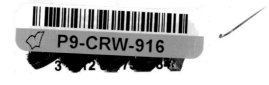

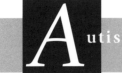

Autism and Early Years Practice

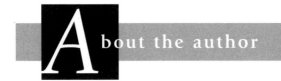

About the author

Kate Wall is Early Childhood Studies Programme Director at Canterbury Christ Church University College. She has worked extensively as a practitioner in early years mainstream and special needs settings. This was initially within primary schools in areas experiencing deprivation, but latterly within preschool provision spanning preschool playgroups, family centres and early years special needs units. Her current work involves teaching undergraduate students as well as leading professional development courses for early years practitioners.

Her knowledge, expertise and skills are further utilised in her work as an author. Kate has published articles in early years journals, chapters in edited works and, of course, her first book Special Needs and Early Years. She has also presented at international conferences.

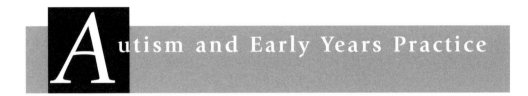

Autism and Early Years Practice

A Guide for Early Years Professionals, Teachers
and Parents

Kate Wall

Paul Chapman Publishing

Paul Chapman Publishing
A SAGE Publications Company
1 Oliver's Yard
55 City Road
London EC1Y 1SP

SAGE Publications Inc.
2455 Teller Road
Thousand Oaks, California 91320

SAGE Publications India Pvt Ltd
B-42, Panchsheel Enclave
New Delhi 100 017

Library of Congress Control Number: 2004100218

A catalogue record for this book is available from the British Library

ISBN 1 4129 0127 8
ISBN 1 4129 0128 6

Typeset by Pantek Arts Ltd, Maidstone, Kent
Printed in Great Britain by T.J. International, Padstow

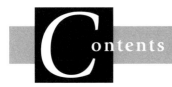

ontents

*F*oreword

On being asked to write a preface for this book, Kate Wall's second in a very short space of time, I was delighted to comply. As in her first book *Special Needs and Early Years: A practitioner's guide*, Kate has provided a rare synthesis of academic rigour, research information and practical knowledge, all linked with her own extensive experience.

As Kate discusses in this book, the field of Early Childhood Education and Care (ECEC) is one in which practitioners are highly committed, dedicated and willing to learn. Generally, they try to do their very best for the children with whom they work. However, Kate also shows that the field has hitherto been neglected in the areas of funding and training. Meanwhile, children whose learning needs are more demanding to staff, who are first and foremost young people (not 'SEN children'), are not having those needs met appropriately. Thankfully, books such as this and Kate's earlier publication are key contributions to the field intended to ameliorate this situation.

It is in their earliest years that children usually begin to gain important understandings about how other people and their worlds 'work'. For example, by around 18 months old, they start to comprehend that those with whom they share their lives, both adults and other children, have different minds from their own, different likes and dislikes, different desires. Along with that comes the ability to understand others' emotions, feelings, meanings and imaginative play. For children with autism such understandings are far more difficult, which makes family and ECEC group life a greater challenge. The parents of autistic children will have experienced fewer 'rewards', such as mutual smiles and protoconversations (early singsong 'chats') with their babies, so they will probably welcome proficient staff who can share their responsibilities and help them see the rewards that their children do offer them.

Autism and Early Years Practice: A Guide for Early Years Professionals, Teachers and Parents, will be an important book for both trainees and existing staff in the ECEC field, whatever their professional backgrounds and titles. As a role model, Kate demonstrates how to be an extended professional – a committed, compassionate, reflective and informed worker, who seeks understanding of children, parents, policy and herself, through observation, theory, research and practice. What is also compelling about such professionals is their strong desire to share their own learning with others in the field, in the hope of improving ECEC for all our children.

Tricia David
Emeritus Professor of Education
Canterbury Christ Church University College
October 2003

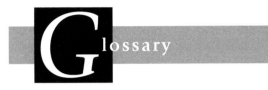
Glossary

ABC	Autism Behaviour Checklist
ADI	Autism Diagnostic Interview
ADOS	Autism Diagnostic Observational Schedule
AIT	Auditory Integration Training
AS	Asperger's syndrome
ASD	Autistic spectrum disorder
BAECE	British Association for early Childhood Education
BOS	Behaviour Observation Scale for Autism
BSE	Behaviour Summarized Evaluation
CARS	Childhood Autism Rating Scale
CD	Creative development
CHAT	Checklist for Autism in Toddlers
CLL	Communication language and literacy
DfES	Department for Education and Skills
DISCO	Diagnostic Interview for Social and Communication Disorders
DRC	Disability Rights Commission
DSM-IV	Diagnostic and Statistical Manual (version 4)
EYDCP	Early Years Development and Childcare Partnership
FC	Facilitated Communication
GP	General practitioner
HIBS	Handicaps and Behaviour Schedule
IBSE	Infant Behavioural Summarized Evaluation
ICD-10	International Classification of Diseases (version 10)
ICT	Information and communications technology
IEP	Individual education plan
IPSEA	Independent Panel for Special Educational Advice
KUW	Knowledge and understanding of the world
LEA	Local education authority
LGA	Local Government Association
MD	Mathematical development
MRC	Medical Research Council
NAS	National Autistic Society
NASEN	National Association for Special Educational Needs
NFER	National Foundation for Educational Research

OFSTED	Office for Standards in Education
PD	Physical development
PDD	Pervasive developmental disorder
PDD-NOS	Pervasive developmental disorder – not otherwise specified
PECS	Picture Exchange Communication System
PL-ADOS	Pre-Linguistic Autism Diagnostic Observation Schedule
PLA	Pre-school Learning Alliance
PPA	Pre-school Playgroups Association
PSE	Personal, social and emotional development
SEN	Special educational needs
SENCO	Special educational needs co-ordinator
SENDA	Special Educational Needs and Disability Discrimination Act
SN	Special needs
TEACCH	The Treatment and Education of Autistic and Related Communication Handicapped Children
WHO	World Health Organization

Terminology

For the purposes of clarity the following terminology will be used throughout this book:

Early years/young children will be considered as aged 0–8 years, but this book will focus predominantly on the under-5s or pre-school children as there is a plethora of information available on children of statutory school age.

Early years provider/provision/setting will refer to any practitioner or establishment providing opportunities and/or support to 0–5-year-old children. This will include pre-school groups, nurseries, nursery classes, childminders, daycare, special needs units/classes/schools and educare groups.

Parents will refer to any person, parent or otherwise, assuming 'parental responsibility' for the child.

Professionals/practitioners refers to any person working with children in any setting, whether or not they hold professional qualifications.

Special educational needs (SEN) will be considered as any difficulties experienced by a child requiring additional or different educational provision to be made.

Special needs (SN) will be considered as those difficulties experienced by a child that do not necessarily result in a special educational need.

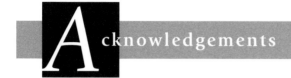

Acknowledgements

My thanks are extended to Estelle, Guy, Pam, Angela, Jo and Carly who have again supported me through the process, for their motivation and support and especially to those who have painstakingly read chapters for me as well. Tricia, who has always inspired me, continues to be a key motivator, and for that I am very grateful. Special thanks must go to those who have given their personal support and encouragement, namely Sam, Tracy and Michael, without whom I would not have completed this work.

This book is dedicated to mum and is also written in memory of Oscar, my 'best buddy'.

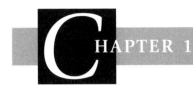

CHAPTER 1

Definitions of autism, common features and relevant legislation

Introduction

In an era of increased inclusion within society in general, early years practitioners are under increasing pressure to accept more and more young children from a range of backgrounds and with a range of individual needs. Current legislation and early years guidance documents also emphasize the importance of providing effectively for all children.

I would suggest that all children have individual needs which change according to their age, circumstances and life events. Some changes will result in a short-term additional need, such as settling in to an early years setting, whilst other needs will be much longer term, such as autism.

This chapter will explore general issues of special needs and early years provision before narrowing the focus to begin unravelling the specific range of autistic spectrum disorders. Through clarifying definitions and identifying the common features, readers will begin their own understanding of 'the autistic world'. This knowledge, combined with the information gained from subsequent chapters will give practitioners increased knowledge of how best to support children with autism and their families. The requirements of current legislation and guidance will be discussed together with the more general definitions of SEN.

Throughout my own working practice with young children with autism I would conclude that whilst such children may have offered me the greatest challenges, they have also given me the greatest rewards, and for that reason they deserve the best that practitioners can offer.

Developments in special needs

Research continues to inform our knowledge and practice and has led to considerable progress over the past century. This progression of knowledge, understanding and awareness of special needs issues within society has led to changes in government policy and, subsequently, legislation.

In the early twentieth century, people experiencing learning difficulties were deemed to be ineducable and terms such as 'idiots' and 'imbeciles' were commonly used to describe them. Sadly, such terms still exist, and are used by a minority today. Within my own working practice I have preferred to discuss 'individual needs' in a more inclusive way as I consider that all children are simply children. Some are tall, some wear glasses, some have autism, but they are all primarily children. If society is developing a more inclusive philosophy then we should rid ourselves of terms such as 'special needs' and 'special educational needs' as our society should be accepting of all and provide for all. If we continue to consider children as having special needs and adapt our provision to accommodate them, we are not demonstrating real inclusion. This issue will continue as long as the government continues to produce separate legislation and guidance documents which segregate or exclude.

However, others may argue that without such separate documentation, effective legislation and provision could not be assured. We therefore continue to work within a 'labelling' framework that can bring its own problems. When welcoming a new child with special needs into our setting we may well have a report informing us of the specific difficulties experienced plus areas of strength and weakness. As practitioners it is then very easy to overlook any additional difficulties the child may be experiencing, but we should always remain vigilant and open-minded to other possibilities. Our expectations should remain high, but realistic, and we should be aware of any possible additional difficulties. For example, children with autism can also experience deafness. The key is to remain open-minded and ensure regular observations and assessments are an ongoing part of our working practice.

Developments in early years provision

In the early twentieth century whilst the value of pre-school provision had been acknowledged in Europe, within the UK there was no statutory pre-school provision for our youngest children. At the start of the twenty-first century we still do not have statutory provision but developments are ongoing and are certainly moving in the right direction. The current government (2003) has initiated a range of important developments such as:

■ Early Years Development and Childcare Partnerships (EYDCPs) and Early Years Development and Childcare Plans from 1998 to work towards providing a free nursery place if parents desire it;

■ National Childcare Strategy to 'ensure all families have access to the childcare which meets their needs' (Internet 1);

■ Early Excellence Centres offering a 'one-stop shop' service for the neighbourhood which integrates education and care provision to offer 'educare'.

As far back as 1929 an education enquiry committee highlighted the differing needs of children under five and therefore the need to offer a separate nursery education, but at that stage no monumental changes were forthcoming. At the start of the Second World War, however, changes began and the 1944 Education Act (Ministry of Education, 1944), which had supported an expansion of nursery education was overtaken by world events. During the war the need for some supported provision became imperative: 'During the Second World War the government supported pre-school provision by way of grants, predominantly to release women to war-related workplaces as the majority of the male workforce was fighting for their country. In addition, the women needed to supplement the poor wages sent home by their husbands.' (Wall, 2003a, p. 5).

After the war pre-school provision continued through a period of expansion but very much at a local, as opposed to national, level and responding very much to local needs. As a result we are now left with a diverse array of provision that varies geographically. There is not, as yet, equality of access for all children and their families to a full range of early years settings.

Additional factors, such as changes in housing policies, also affected the future for our youngest children. For example, in the 1950s and 1960s high-rise flats were built in many large towns and cities throughout the country. This resulted in many families with young children being segregated from their local communities for considerable periods of time, thus limiting social and educational opportunities for both parents and children alike.

> **Illustrative example 1.1**
>
> A single mother with three children aged 2, 3 and 6 lives on the twelfth floor of a block of flats in a large inner city development area. The 6-year-old attends school from Monday to Friday between 9 a.m. and 3 p.m., the 3-year-old attends the local pre-school group three times a week from 9.30 a.m. to 12 noon and the toddler attends mother and toddler group two afternoons a week from 1.30 p.m. to 3 p.m.
>
> With a double buggy to manage in the lift (when working) the practicalities of coping with so many trips in any one week are considerable. The mother could be forgiven on a wet and cold wintery day for not taking the younger children to their settings regularly. This of course does not take into account the need to go to the supermarket, the health centre, the post office, the bank and so on. It is not an easy task, which is certain to place considerable pressure on the mother and, indirectly, the children.

In the 1960s the playgroup movement became firmly established in the UK. Responding to local gaps in provision, playgroups predominantly opened in village halls and community centres offering part-time social play sessions to local 3- and 4-year-olds. Playgroups were normally run by a committee of parents and local early years professionals, and the sessions used rotas of mothers and volunteers, some of whom may have had early years or teaching qualifications. Over subsequent years the Pre-school Playgroups Association (PPA) evolved (now the Pre-School Learning Alliance, PLA) which initiated local networks and training for playgroup workers as well as campaigning for the early years. Playgroups have since been renamed pre-schools.

Since the 1960s we have seen the development in family centres, funded by education, social services, jointly or by voluntary organizations; early excellence centres; and four-year-olds being accepted into nursery classes attached to and funded by schools.

The resultant range of early years provision is considerable and is well documented (Pugh, 2001; Wall, 2003a), but would include:

1. Statutory services

    a. primary schools – providing for children aged 4 to 11 years

    b. nursery schools and classes

    c. day nurseries and family centres

    d. home based support

2. Private services:

   a. childminders

   b. private nursery schools

   c. private day nurseries

   d. workplace nurseries

   e. nannies/au pairs

   f. out-of-school clubs

3. Voluntary services:

   a. playgroups (pre-schools)

   b. groups affiliated to charitable organisations. (Wall, 2003a, p. 10)

This diversity is not necessarily consistent with equality of access for all. It will, as previously indicated, vary according to what is available in each neighbourhood. This variance should be further unified in the future.

Autism

Autism, like many other conditions or disorders, can affect people in a variety of ways, but is a lifelong developmental disability. I would suggest that unless practitioners have a good knowledge and understanding of autism then they may not be able to provide appropriately, and may inadvertently compound a child's difficulty through lack of knowledge.

What is autism?

As a developmental disability autism can affect children, and adults, in a variety of ways and in varying degrees. Children with autism may be referred to as 'aloof' or 'withdrawn' as they appear disinterested in the world around them. Unlike other children the lack of desire to be part of so-called 'normal' everyday life presents practitioners and parents with an immediate barrier – how to access the world of the child to enable support and appropriate provision. If a child does not want to interact with anyone and only wishes to play with a box of toy trains, then how can we begin to plan to ensure progress?

In 1943 Leo Kanner presented a clinical paper highlighting the key features of children with 'early infantile autism', thus naming the condition, which previously had been accepted as an extreme mental disorder, considered by some to be the result of very poor mothering resulting in the child withdrawing into him/herself.

Possibly one of the first recorded incidences of autism came at around the turn of the nineteenth century. A boy of about 12 years, later named Victor, was discovered in woodland near Aveyron in France, apparently having lived in the wild for most of his young life. In 1799 he was caught and taken to Jean Mark Gaspard Itard in Paris who began a period of observation which was methodically recorded and clearly indicated classic autistic features. Itard was fascinated by Victor's ability to focus on familiar things for long periods of time and despite having no prior experience, proceeded to work with Victor, using Victor's strengths to guide his interventions. Victor's social behaviour progressed considerably despite the fact that he did not speak, and he learned to communicate in an alternative, non-verbal manner. He also became able to function more appropriately, in human company. This, compared to the swaying, biting and scratching young boy that first appeared from the woods was enormous progress for its time. Itard had also been teaching Seguin, a student, and passed on his findings and knowledge from his experiences with Victor. Seguin was influential in the later work of Montessori.

Returning to Kanner's work, his article recorded the outcomes of 11 case histories, concluding that whilst some of the characteristics demonstrated by the children could be closely linked to existing syndromes or conditions, there was a clear indication of a separate and unique condition emerging. These characteristics included:

■ lack of desire to communicate verbally;

■ echolalic verbal utterances;

■ fear in strange or unexpected situations;

■ lack of imaginative play activities;

■ repetitive behaviours demonstrated.

Kanner also concluded that for some children the condition, or at least the predisposing conditions, were evident from birth whilst for other children the characteristics would not emerge until 2 or 3 years of age, and often in a regressive manner, that is, they appeared to develop skills which later disappeared. Wing (1976) suggests that Kanner's reference to early infantile autism is 'inappropriate':

> Kanner's own preferred name 'early infantile autism' is not entirely
> appropriate since, in some cases an otherwise typical syndrome has

developed during the second or third year of life. 'Early childhood autism' is probably not the most satisfactory term, since it does not carry the implication of an inevitable onset from birth and it does suggest that the autism is 'maximal' in early life and may improve later. (p. 21)

Some would extend such a debate to suggest the term 'autism' itself is misleading, as Bleuler (1919) had identified autism as 'one of the fundamental symptoms of schizophrenia' (Wing, 1976, p. 11). Wing continues to highlight a key difference between Bleuler's and Kanner's usages of the term, describing Bleuler's understanding of those with autism as demonstrating 'an active withdrawal from contact with the world' (p. 11), whereas Kanner's understanding outlined an 'inability to relate'. This difference is still significant today as our understanding of autistic behaviours focuses on the lack of desire or perceived need to interact with others, more in line with Kanner's work. This was also discussed by Rutter and Schopler (1978).

Asperger's syndrome

Following Kanner's paper in 1943, Hans Asperger highlighted a similar condition, Asperger's syndrome, whereby children and adults demonstrating many features of autism appear quite able intellectually. Siegel (1996) summarized a fundamental difference between autism and Asperger's syndrome: 'most AS individuals have more mild impairments, higher IQs (especially higher verbal IQs), and a better ability to adapt than most autistic people' (p. 113). However, as Asperger's work and findings evolved at a time of war, little was known about it until the early 1990s when Frith published a translation of Asperger's paper, and since then the term has been used more widely.

There are many adults today who have only in adulthood been diagnosed as having Asperger's syndrome. Able to attend mainstream schools and to secure later employment, these adults may have difficulties with, or feel uncomfortable with, social situations and often demonstrate precision, or repetitive behaviour patterns, in many areas of their lives. Attwood (1998) succinctly highlights the common features of Asperger's syndrome: 'A lack of social skills, limited ability to have a reciprocal conversation and an intense interest in a particular subject are core features of this syndrome' (p. 13).

Defining autism

Perhaps settling on one definition of autism is seeking the impossible as a vast array of definitions have been offered over the years. However, three classic features, which should all occur, arise in every definition and are often combined with repetitive and stereotypical behaviours. The impairments are in social interaction, communication and imagination.

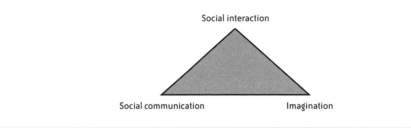

Figure 1.1 The triad of impairments

Impairments in one or more of the above areas would not in itself warrant a diagnosis of autism. The final consideration is that the features must be present before the child reaches the age of 3. These three characteristics of autism are generally known as the triad of impairments (see Figure 1.1).

Over the past 20 years, as more knowledge has been gained from research and provision for children with autism has progressed, it has been common to hear of the 'autistic spectrum' (see Figure 1.2) extending from severe autism through to Asperger's syndrome. What should always be remembered is that no two children with autism will present the same characteristics to the same degree, just as no two children are the same. The important key is for practitioners to increase their knowledge and understanding of autism so that children with autism that attend their settings can be supported and provided for in a way that will enable them to work towards their full potential. As with all children, talking to parents, observing the child, identifying their strengths, likes and dislikes, combined with knowledge and understanding of autistic spectrum disorders, will all inform planning and respond to the child's individual needs. Effective planning related to the individual needs of the child is the key for providing for children with autism, and even the child diagnosed with severe autism can benefit considerably, thus enhancing future opportunities and moving them away from the severe autism diagnosis on the autistic spectrum.

The current government guidance document *Autistic Spectrum Disorders: Good Practice Guidelines* (DfES/DoH, 2002) offers the following description of autistic spectrum disorders:

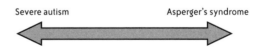

Figure 1.2 The autistic spectrum

> *Autistic spectrum disorder is a relatively new term to denote the fact that there are a number of subgroups within the spectrum of autism. There are differences between the subgroups and further work is required on defining the criteria, but all children with an ASD share a triad of impairments in their ability to:*

> ■ *Understand and use non-verbal and verbal communication*

> ■ *Understand social behaviour which affects their ability to interact with children and adults*

> ■ *Think and behave flexibly – which may be shown in restricted, obsessional or repetitive activities. (s. 2.1)*

Perhaps a more accessible definition is offered by the Treatment and Education of Autistic and Communication Handicapped Children programme (TEACCH).

> *Autism is a lifelong developmental disability that prevents individuals from properly understanding what they see, hear and otherwise sense. This results in severe problems of social relationships, communication and behaviour. Individuals with autism have to painstakingly learn normal patterns of speech and communication, and appropriate ways to relate to people, objects and events in a similar manner to those who have had a stroke. (Internet 2)*

Prevalence of autism

Figures relating to the prevalence of autism vary, and research documents and projects have repeatedly tried to produce the most recent and accurate figures. However, the fact that autism has become increasingly better understood over the past 20 years has resulted in an increase in such figures. This should not necessarily be interpreted as an increase in the prevalence of autism in children, more as an indication of increased knowledge and understanding.

Prevalence figures are further complicated by identifying those with classic autism, or Asperger's syndrome or even pervasive developmental disorder – not otherwise specified (PDD-NOS). It can be difficult to discriminate between autism and PDD-NOS as many similar characteristics may appear. It therefore depends on the skills of the professional undertaking the diagnosis. Siegel (1996) summarizes the key differences:

> *Generally, PDD, NOS can be thought of as essentially constituting a less severe, or less fully symptomatic form of autism. Research studies have shown that autism and PDD, NOS often have the same profile of symptoms but that the symptoms tend to be less numerous and less severe in the child diagnosed with PDD, NOS. (p.15)*

Considering England only, Lotter (1967) presented the rate for autism at that time as 4.4 per 10,000 people, whilst just over ten years later Wing and Gould (1978) presented a rate of 4.9 per 10,000 people. More recently, the National Autistic Society (NAS) suggested that across the whole spectrum of autistic disorders the rate is 90 per 10,000. All studies agree that the incidence in boys is greater than that of girls, but again no clear figure is offered. A reasonable average would be to consider the ratio as 1:4, girls to boys. For practitioners, the reality is that they will be likely to meet several children with autism during their professional career.

Signs of autism

Some young children with autism will have developed along accepted developmental paths in the first 24–36 months of their life, but often speech development may have been a little delayed (which is not uncommon in young children, and especially in boys). Similarly a child's social skills could be delayed. Noticeable changes may then arise and initially these changes may be slow to appear, but at some point parents will begin to see elements of regression such as:

- ■ new words may be used by a child a few times and then disappear;

- ■ the child begins to repeat words, phrases or the ends of sentences spoken to them in a 'parrot-like' fashion (echolalia);

- ■ the child becomes more withdrawn, preferring solitary play;

- ■ the type of play becomes less imaginative and more repetitive, e.g. only playing with six cars and persistently lining them up;

- ■ increased fear of new situations and people;

- ■ resistance to change in routine;

- ■ the child may no longer give direct eye contact but look out of the corner of his/her eye at people or objects (peripheral vision);

- the child may develop an obsessional fascination with one object, e.g. light switches or doors;

- lack of fear or awareness of danger;

- sensitivity to some sensory stimuli, e.g. refusing to eat 'lumpy' food, averse to loud noises.

For those children who demonstrate autistic tendencies from birth, the following signs are indicative of an autistic spectrum disorder:

- baby does not develop eye contact, appearing disinterested when adults or objects approach;

- difficulty with sleeping or perfect 'sleeper';

- prolonged periods of extreme placidness;

- lack of babbling noises or sounds;

- no desire to be picked up;

- may seem agitated if cuddled.

However, one or more of these signs could mean acceptable, but delayed, development or be indicative of another disorder. For example, a placid baby may seem a bonus for many parents, but if the child does not develop babbling noise then this may be a sign of a hearing impairment. For such reasons a diagnosis of an autistic spectrum disorder in the first year of life is considered inappropriate.

During the period from 12 to 24 months these tendencies then become more developed and often it is the parents who notice their child's unusual patterns of behaviour. Signs at this stage could include:

- lack of interest in exploratory, exciting play;

- the child seeming comfortable in his/her own world with no apparent need for any interaction with other children or adults;

- being difficult to understand. The child may appear distressed but parents are unable to ascertain the reasons as no meaningful speech has evolved;

- unusual movements that may occur, such as hand-flapping, rocking or placing hands over ears;

- play being repetitive and apparently unimaginative;

- no development of pretend play;

- still resisting changes in routine and fearful of new situations;

- sensitivity to some stimuli becoming more pronounced;

- inability to interpret gestures or facial expressions;

- inability to understand language other than literally, e.g. 'Jump in the bath' can be interpreted by the child as a request to jump up and down in the bath, whereas the adult simply means 'It's time to have a bath'.

At this point this produces many difficulties for the family and friends as the child's, as yet undiagnosed, autistic behaviours may resemble that of a misbehaving child whose parents are incapable of controlling him/her. Such situations can be severely compounded by the reactions and comments of members of the public. Issues relating to the families of children with autism will be further explored in Chapter 2.

Characteristics of autism

If we reflect on the triad of impairments presented earlier (Figure 1.1) we can begin to translate the signs of autism into the three areas of difficulty indicative of an autistic spectrum disorder. This should help clarify the characteristics of this disorder, although practitioners should remember that these key characteristics will vary in intensity from child to child:

1. Social interaction:

    (a) Avoids eye contact.

    (b) Lack of desire to interact or play with other children or adults.

    (c) Appears oblivious to the world around.

    (d) Is not interested in being picked up, played with or cuddled.

    (e) Lack of co-operative or parallel play.

    (f) Lack of desire to establish relationships and friendships.

    (g) Unable to interpret or understand people's feelings and emotions.

    (h) Does not respond to affection or being touched or appears to overreact.

2. Social communication (speech, language and non-verbal communication):

    (a) Lack of useful language.

    (b) Lack of desire to communicate with others around them.

    (c) Echolalia.

    (d) Inability to understand non-verbal communication such as gestures and facial expression.

    (e) Inability to understand the process of conversation.

    (f) If speech develops, it will be delayed and may demonstrate unusual speech, unusual or monotonous tone and/or patterns of speech.

    (g) May talk about a topic incessantly and at inappropriate times.

    (h) May be able to use language appropriately in one situation but be unable to transfer the language into an alternative situation.

3. Imagination:

    (a) Lack of imaginative play.

    (b) Play may be rigid, stereotypical and repetitive.

    (c) Resistance to participate in imaginative play situations.

    (d) Repetitive and/or obsessive behaviours.

    (e) Difficulties and anxieties coping with changes to routines.

In addition to the characteristics above, the following may be observed:

- repetitive movements such as hand-flapping, rocking or covering ears or eyes;

- unusual response to stimuli. Children with autism may be oversensitive or undersensitive to some sensory stimuli. Examples would include: refusal to eat 'lumpy' food or combined foods such as sandwiches; aversion to common noises such as a dishwasher or vacuum cleaner; apparent lack of awareness of cold and heat. (This raises particular issues of possible danger.);

- difficulties with poor or delayed motor co-ordination – gross body and/or fine/motor;

- unusual responses to 'normal' situations;

- self-harming or inappropriate behaviour, such as overaggressive play;

- erratic sleeping patterns;

- a skill that the child excels at – usually in art, knowledge of a film, music or mathematics. Children with such an exceptional skill are known as 'autistic savants'.

Illustrative example 1.2

Toby arrives at your setting

Toby is 3 and is awaiting an appointment with the local consultant paediatrician for a full developmental assessment. The health visitor has expressed concerns regarding his lack of verbal communication and withdrawn nature. The report given to the setting suggests that Toby demonstrates 'autistic type tendencies'.

When Toby first enters the setting he is screaming and flapping his hands. Once inside he spots the home corner and runs towards it, opening and shutting each and every door repeatedly and noisily. A member of staff goes to say hello to him but he ignores her and continues to bang the cupboard doors. Other children in the setting are uneasy about the noise from the door-banging and the non-verbal noises Toby is making.

Toby's mum speaks to the setting manager saying she is so relieved that Toby has been accepted into the setting as she is desperate for any help she can be given. She hands over Toby's cup as he refuses to drink from any other and will become distressed if encouraged to use another cup. Mum also provides his own snack for breaktime, as he has a range of food intolerances, plus his favourite toy train which he needs to be able to access at all times.

At breaktime Toby refuses to sit with the group and screams throughout singing time.

Consider the following:

1. Support needed for Toby's mum?

2. How are you going to support Toby's settling in period?

3. How are you going to begin to involve Toby in other activities?

▶

4. How will you deal with the reactions of other children in the setting and their parents?

5. Do you feel your staff have sufficient understanding of autism to respond to his needs effectively?

6. Who would you contact for additional support addressing Toby's needs?

As can be seen, this scenario raises a whole range of important issues that must be thought through and addressed to ensure Toby's needs are met. It is a summary of my first encounter with a young child with autism and, at that time, I was at a loss as to how to provide for this little boy. I was aware that my knowledge and understanding of autism should be extended considerably, and rapidly, if I was going to continue working effectively with him.

From Illustrative example 1.2 we can see that Toby's difficulties were unfamiliar to the staff of the setting and this raises a key point for all practitioners. We cannot be experts in every type of disorder, syndrome and difficulty a child can experience but, as long as we are prepared to recognize this and improve our own knowledge and understanding, we will continue to provide the best opportunities we can for the children we work with.

Causes of autism

Research is ongoing to discover the causes of autism, but as yet, no definitive answer can be offered. Genetic factors and problems with brain development are, however, believed to be closely linked. The following explanation is offered by the TEACCH programme:

> *Autism is a brain disorder, present from birth, which affects the way the brain uses information. The cause of autism is still unknown. Some research suggests a physical problem affecting those parts of the brain that process language and information coming in from the senses. There may be some imbalance of certain chemicals in the brain. Genetic factors may sometimes be involved. Autism may indeed result from a combination of 'several' causes. (Internet 2)*

Some professionals support the discrimination between classic autism (from birth) and regressive autism, which develops at a later stage, commonly between the ages of 18 and 24 months.

Similar or linked disorders

As previously discussed, autism can include signs and symptoms that are also indicative of other disorders and conditions, hence the need for thorough and detailed diagnostic procedures by highly qualified professionals. The following conditions should provide a useful summary for practitioners and can be split into two categories:

1   Conditions within the autistic spectrum.

    (a) *Asperger's syndrome.* Difficulties with social interactions but not normally delayed in speech and language development. Children with Asperger's syndrome demonstrate normal or high levels of intelligence and are thus at the more able end of the autistic spectrum.

    (b) *PDD-NOS.* Pervasive developmental disorder – not otherwise specified does not have a clear definition and is explored when difficulties allied to autistic difficulties are present but no other explanation can be offered. The key difference is that with PDD-NOS the autistic symptoms are not as well developed or not all the features of an autistic diagnosis are present. It may be that a diagnosis of autism is sought or suggested but that with detailed and thorough assessment, not all autistic criteria are met.

    (c) *Childhood disintegrative disorder or Heller's syndrome.* As the name suggests childhood disintegrative disorder can be diagnosed when a child who has followed the expected developmental path appears to regress, or their childhood appears to 'disintegrate'. However, unlike regressive autism, the regression often does not begin until the child is 3 years or over. The discrete differences between the two conditions are still under research to clarify the issues and thus aid and inform diagnostic procedures. Seizures often form a part of this condition.

    (d) *Rett's syndrome.* Rett's syndrome only affects girls and is suggested as affecting only 1 per 10,000 children (Trevarthen et al., 1998). Again a pattern of expected development occurs, but only in the first few months of life. This is then followed by a period of regression affecting speech and language, social, behavioural and physical development. All children with Rett's syndrome develop severe or profound learning difficulties. Due to the similarities between Rett's and autism many children can benefit from interventions and strategies used to support children with autism. Again care should be taken with the diagnostic process, as indicated by Siegel (1996): 'Between the second and fifth or sixth year of life, when Rett's syndrome is usually first diagnosed, the girl may also meet diagnostic criteria for Autism or PDD because of a marked lack of social relatedness and the presence of other features of autism' (p. 22). Siegel suggests that this social relatedness often fades over subsequent years and adolescents can develop more appropriate social skills.

2   Conditions linked with autism but not within the autistic spectrum.

   (a) *Childhood schizophrenia*. For many years autism and schizophrenia were considered to be similar, overlapping conditions. However studies in the 1960s and 1970s concluded the debate by highlighting a number of significant differences between schizophrenia and autism. Most importantly, hallucinations, unreasonable and inappropriate behaviour combined with normal development of speech and the lack of learning disabilities are a few of the key indicators of schizophrenia which are not usually associated with autism. However it is possible, although rare, for a child to have schizophrenia and autism.

   (b) *Landau-Kleffner syndrome*. Similarly, children with Landau-Kleffner syndrome also appear to develop according to expected pathways, but a later regression between 3 and 8 years of age affects speech and language development, and is usually preceded by the onset of seizures. Characteristics include: affected language comprehension and expressive speech plus behavioural difficulties. The following summarizes the possible confusion with autism: 'Some children have episodes of very abnormal 'autistic type behaviour' with symptoms such as avoidance of contact with family and friends (avoidance of eye contact is common) extreme pickiness over food, very disturbed sleep, attacks of rage and aggression, insensitivity to pain, bizarre and inappropriate and repetitive play' (Internet 3).

(c) *Specific language disorders*. Young children with specific speech and language disorders may also experience difficulties in social skills and social interactions caused by the effects of the speech and language disorder. For example, a young child with an expressive language difficulty may prefer to remain silent or use limited speech to avoid being misunderstood by others around him/her. Clearly this can also affect their emotional development. For such reasons a diagnosis of autism may be considered but through detailed assessment, based on a speech and language therapy assessment, an appropriate diagnosis should follow.

(d) *William's syndrome*. William's syndrome affects only 1 in 20,000 and is present from birth (Internet 4). Facial features are characterized by a small nose and chin, a wide mouth with full lips and apparent swelling surrounding the eyes. In addition, teeth are undersized and have gaps between them. Babies with William's syndrome often have difficulties feeding due to poor muscle tone, and difficulties with sucking and swallowing. They also suffer from more severe colic than other babies. Children with William's syndrome also experience delayed development (including speech and language problems) and learning difficulties; however, many will develop speech as they mature but this may appear as the repetitive use of language.

(e) *Prader-Willi syndrome*. Prader-Willi syndrome, which affects boys and girls (estimated prevalence 1:12,000–15,000 (Internet 5) is defined as: 'a complex genetic disorder that typically causes low muscle tone, short stature, incomplete sexual development, cognitive disabilities, problem behaviours, and a chronic feeling of hunger that can lead to excessive eating and life-threatening obesity' (Internet 5). Caused by a chromosome disorder children with Prader-Willi syndrome will be delayed in expected developmental milestones from birth. The feeding difficulties experienced as a baby will be replaced later with a desire to eat constantly, often leading to chronic obesity which can be life threatening.

(f) *Fragile X syndrome*. Fragile X is a chromosomal abnormality which has been linked with autism and, generally speaking, the effects on boys are significantly greater that those on girls. Cumine, Leach and Stephenson (2000) highlight the link with autism: 'Fragile X features most prominently in its association with autism, in that 26% per cent of the Fragile X population children with severe learning difficulties also have autism' (p. 27). The behavioural characteristics of Fragile X include hand-flapping, 'autistic type behaviours' (Internet 6) poor eye contact, sensitivity to sound and touch plus poor attention span. In addition boys with Fragile X syndrome will experience severe learning difficulties, whilst girls will experience moderate difficulties with learning. Physical characteristics include large, prominent ears and an elongated face.

(g) *Angelman syndrome*. Also caused by a chromosome defect wherein some similarities can be seen between Angelman syndrome and autism, however, children with Angelman syndrome invariably have severe learning difficulties. Sometimes this syndrome is referred to as 'Happy Puppet' syndrome as children present with a smiling face and hold their arms out stiffly rather like a puppet.

The preceding list of disorders linked with autism, and/or those that sometimes appear with autism in children is considerable but not exhaustive. It should give practitioners an understanding of those more frequently presented.

Legislation and guidance

Developments in special needs legislation

Although in current legislation practitioners work within definitions and labels of 'special needs', 'special educational needs' and 'children in need', I would suggest that whilst such terms may support appropriate provision, they may also give rise to difficulties. As long as we continue to regard special needs provision as separate and discrete from mainstream provision, which includes the government's continued production of separate documentation for special needs, then we are not offering an inclusive service. Separate legislation and guidance excludes, not includes. If we consider the work we undertake with children with autism, we observe and assess their strengths, likes and dislikes and use this information to inform our planning and interventions. This is not different practice for children with special needs but positive and effective early years practice for *all* children.

Historically, developments in special needs legislation have seen the most rapid changes during the past 25 years. During the nineteenth and early twentieth centuries those with special needs were usually regarded as ineducable. Through the 1920s and 1930s Freud's work was becoming established and renowned. Linking adult behaviours and feelings to experiences in early childhood offered explanations for some difficulties experienced by adults and began to inform society that such people were not 'imbeciles' but were suffering from illness.

In 1970 the Education (Handicapped Children) Act (DES, 1970) was the impetus for the establishment of an increased range of special schools for children with:

- moderate learning difficulties (MLD);

- severe learning difficulties (SLD);

- severely subnormal difficulties (SSD) (Wall, 2003a, p. 12).

In 1978, possibly the most significant document to date was produced, the Warnock Report (DES, 1978). Reviewing all current provision for children with special educational needs the report's recommendations were carried through into the 1981 Education Act (DES, 1981). Within the Act were revised definitions of special educational needs for practitioners to work within.

The Children Act of 1989 evolved to consolidate previous public and private laws regarding children with the key principle of the welfare of the child being 'paramount' at all times. The Children Act relates predominantly to issues surrounding families and children (including a review of child protection procedures) plus registration requirements for all registered early years providers (DoH, 1989).

The Code of Practice (DfEE, 1994) followed the 1993 Education Act (DfEE, 1993) and detailed the responsibilities of all local education authorities (LEAs) and education providers regarding identification, assessment (within a five-staged process), reviews, statements of SEN and the introduction of the special educational needs co-ordinator (SENCO). This was the first governmental guidance document to include requirements for children under 5 years of age.

Although not specifically relating to special needs provision, the Nursery Education and Grant Maintained Schools Act of 1996 (DfEE, 1996) is pertinent to the current discussion as it relates to the introduction of the Nursery Voucher Scheme, giving parents vouchers which were redeemable at a range of local pre-school settings. This was the first legislation for pre-school providers which included the inspection of settings according to criteria defined within the Act. As opposed to the existing social services inspections, which predominantly examined issues of health and safety, the Office for Standards in Education (Ofsted) inspections considered issues relating to the quality of provision offered.

Current legislation and guidance

The most recent legislation is the Special Educational Needs and Disability Discrimination Act or SENDA (DfES, 2001a) which was followed by the *Special Educational Needs Code of Practice* (DfES, 2001b). The five-staged approach to identification and assessment from the 1994 Code of Practice has been replaced by Early Years Action and Early Years Action Plus for children under 5 years old, and School Action and School Action Plus for those in Key Stage 1 and above. The Code of Practice states that:

> Once practitioners have identified that a child has special educational
> needs, the setting should intervene through Early Years Action. If the
> intervention does not enable the child to make satisfactory progress the
> SENCO may need to seek advice and support from external agencies. These
> forms of intervention are referred to (below) as Early Years Action Plus.
> (DfES, 2001b, s. 4:11)

The Code of Practice includes new chapters on identification and assessment and, for the first time, a whole chapter on provision in early years settings. In addition there is a strong emphasis on provision occurring within effective multidisciplinary networks, thus providing a 'seamless' service to young children and their families. Other initiatives within the Code include a stronger influence on effective partnerships with parents and involving the children in their own assessments and reviews.

The definition of special educational needs within the current Code of Practice that practitioners are working with states that:

> Children have special educational needs if they have a learning difficulty
> which calls for special educational provision to be made for them.
>
> Children have a learning difficulty if they:
>
> (a) Have a significantly greater difficulty in learning than the majority of
>   children of the same age; or

> (b) *Have a disability which prevents or hinders them from making use of educational facilities of a kind generally provided for children of the same age in schools within the area of the local education authority;*
>
> (c) *Are under compulsory school age and fall within the definition at (a) or (b) above or would do so if special educational provision was not made for them. (DfES, 2001a, s. 1:3)*

Since the publication of the Code of Practice, organizations such as the National Association for Special Educational Needs (NASEN) have highlighted possible difficulties or limitations of the Code, such as the lack of administration and planning time for SENCOs and the need for training and funding to ensure the code is implemented fully and to the positive benefit of all children with special educational needs.

The SENDA also updates issues of disability discrimination and the Disability Rights Commission (DRC) has issued their own Disability Discrimination Act *Draft Code of Practice* for Schools. This document guides settings on 'preventing discrimination against disabled people in their access to education' (DRC, 2001, p. 7) and suggests two duties that settings should take heed of to ensure that pupils are not discriminated against:

- not to treat disabled pupils less favourably; and

- to make reasonable adjustments to avoid putting disabled pupils at a substantial disadvantage (ibid. p. 15).

As well as the Code of Practice the DfES has produced several additional guidance documents to support practitioners:

- *Special Educational Needs Toolkit* (DfES, 2001c);

- *Inclusive Schooling: Children with Special Educational Needs* (DfES, 2001d);

- *Access to Education for Children with Medical Needs* (DfES, 2001e);

- *Autistic Spectrum Disorders: Good Practice Guidance* (DfES/DoH, 2002).

The latter will clearly be of great interest to those working with children with autism and offers practitioners two guidance booklets: *01 Guidance on Autistic Spectrum Disorders* and *02 Pointers to Good Practice*. These will be referred to in later chapters.

Clearly the government is committed to providing effective provision for all young children with special needs but it could be suggested that the publication of more and detailed documentation does not on its own ensure effective provision. Such documents take time to read, assimilate and disseminate to all staff members and, thus, training for practitioners should be a priority.

Summary

Within this chapter the developments in early years provision have been examined to highlight the range of diverse settings available to parents of young children. Sadly the range of accessible settings within any one locality will probably differ from neighbouring localities and 'thus' equity of access to provision is still an issue. The developments within special needs provision were also explored and highlighted the transition from separate special school settings to the current more inclusive system in which practitioners are expected to be able to provide for increasing numbers of children with special needs. The issues of training and funding were identified as concerns if we wish to ensure that all early years practitioners can provide effectively for the individual needs of all children.

Autistic spectrum disorders were then explored to offer the reader increased understanding and knowledge of this range of disorders. A brief history of autism and Asperger's syndrome followed, to highlight the main differences and how they fitted into the autistic spectrum. The triad of impairments, indicative of autism was identified and definitions of autism were offered. The signs of autism in young children should also support practitioner knowledge and were linked back to the three areas of impairment that form the triad. The example of Toby was introduced to relate the listing of signs and characteristics to the reality of the children that we may work with. A range of disorders that are similar to or linked to autism were outlined to highlight crucial issues for diagnosis but also to remind practitioners that we should always remain open-minded. The rather brief résumé of legislation and guidance summarized the current situation, showing that the move towards increasing inclusion, whilst a positive move for children with any special need, should be supported by training for all practitioners to ensure that all children's needs can, and will, be met in our early years settings.

Key issues

■ *Practitioners may need to increase their knowledge and understanding of autism to provide effectively for children with autistic spectrum disorders.*

■ *Effective provision for children with autism is not different practice but positive and effective early years practice for all children.*

■ *Current legislation and guidance covers special needs, special educational needs, providing for children on the autistic spectrum, disability discrimination and human rights.*

■ *Within the current move towards increased inclusion there are still key issues to be addressed.*

Some suggestions for discussion

Item 1

Initiate a discussion of training of all those working in your setting. Consider the following:

■ knowledge of current legislation and guidance;

■ knowledge and skills to provide for the needs of all the children within your setting;

■ knowledge and understanding of autistic spectrum disorders;

■ abilities to provide for the needs of children with autism in your setting.

Item 2

In the light of the above discussion, review training needs for the future.

Item 3

Focus on one child with autism that you either are currently working with or have worked with previously and consider:

■ Do you feel you have sufficient understanding of their difficulties to provide appropriately?

■ Does your planning respond directly to their needs?

■ Could improved knowledge of autism improve your provision for the child?

📖 Suggested further reading

Department for Education and Science (DfES) (2001). *Special Educational Needs Code of Practice*. Nottingham: DfES.

Department for Education and Science/Department of Health (DfES/DoH). (2002). *Autistic Spectrum Disorders: Good Practice Guidance*. Nottingham: DfES.

Trevarthen, C., Aitken, K., Papoudi, D. and Robarts, J. (1998). *Children with Autism: Diagnosis and Interventions to Meet Their Needs*. London: Jessica Kingsley, Chapters 2, 3 and 4.

Wall, K. (2003). *Special Needs and Early Years: A Practitioner's Guide*. London: Sage, Chapter 1.

Useful contacts – some examples of supporting agencies

Advisory Centre for Education (ACE)
Unit 1c Aberdeen Studios, 22–24 Highbury Grove, London N5 2DQ

☎ 0207 354 8318   🖥 www.ace-ed.org.uk

Autism Independent UK (formerly the Society for the Treatment of the Autistically Handicapped)
199–205 Blandford Ave, Kettering, Northants NN16 9AT

☎ 01536 523274   🖥 www.autismuk.com

British Association for Early Childhood Education (BAECE)
136 Cavell Street, London E1 2JA

☎ 0207 539 5400   🖥 www.early-education.org.uk

Disability Rights Commission (DRC)
Freepost MID 02164, Stratford-upon-Avon, CV37 9BR

☎ 08457 622 633   🖥 www.drc.org.uk

Independent Panel for Special Educational Advice (IPSEA)
6 Carlow Mews, Woodbridge, Suffolk IP12 1DH

☎ 01394 382814   🖥 www.ipsea.org.uk

National Association for Special Educational Needs (NASEN)
4–5 Amber Business Village, Amber Close, Amington, Tamworth B77 4RP

☎ 01827 311500   🖥 www.nasen.org.uk

National Autistic Society
393 City Road, London EC1V 1NG
☎ 0207 833 2299   🖳 www.nas.org.uk

National Children's Bureau, Early Childhood Unit,
8 Wakley Street, London EC1V 7QE
☎ 020 7843 6000   🖳 www.ncb.org.uk

Network 81 (for parents of children with special educational needs)
1–7 Woodfield Terrace, Stansted, Essex CM24 8AJ
☎ 0800 770 3263   🖳 www.network81.co.uk

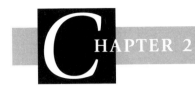

CHAPTER 2

Families of children with autism

Introduction

Early years practitioners are now expected to provide for more children with a diverse range of special needs than perhaps ever before. To provide effectively for children with special needs requires expertise and skills combined with knowledge of not only the child's disorder or condition, but also current legislation and guidance relating to special needs provision. Considerable time is now devoted to observing children, assessing their needs, planning activities, writing individual education plans (IEPs), evaluating progress, writing progress reviews, working with other agencies and working with parents. Yet how much time is spent reflecting on the needs of individual family members?

In this chapter the perspectives of families of children with autism will be explored, identifying particular issues relating to parents, grandparents and siblings. When combined with a discussion of the range of influencing factors on the development of children, the importance of this area will be highlighted. This will be further developed through a discussion of the importance of positive partnerships with parents and effective multi-agency working systems to support families.

Children and families

The days of two-parent families with the stereotypical 2.4 children, living within a community that is also shared by many extended family members is long past. Although some families may still exist in this way, they are likely to be in the minority. Family structures themselves have changed over the years and practitioners should be aware of the effects of a variety of family structures the children they work with will be living in. In addition, some thought can be given to the effects of the following family structures on very young children:

- Conjugal nuclear – a man and a woman are married and living together with their children.

- Non-conjugal nuclear – a man and woman are living together with their children but are not legally married.

- Lone parent – a man or a woman living apart from their partner, possibly as the result of death or separation.

- Reconstituted – one lone parent living with another lone parent or a single adult.

- Extended – more than one generation of a family living together.

- Gay/lesbian – two gay or lesbian adults living together as partners.

- Adoptive families – two adults living together (generally married) who have adopted children.

- Care homes – children living in a local authority community home due to a range of reasons prohibiting them from living in their family home.

Within any of these family structures the responsible adults, and therefore the children, may be affected by factors such as grief and/or loss, financial difficulties, unemployment, poor housing, limited support networks and access to transport. In circumstances such as redundancy the resulting effects on the adults could create stress and tension and, whilst there may be attempts to keep the children distanced from the extent of the difficulties, even young children can be severely affected either in the short or the longer term. Whilst practitioners may not be able directly to support the family's difficulties, awareness and understanding can inform them regarding their provision for the child. More sensitive care and perhaps more time for adult attention on a one-to-one basis may help to reduce the negative effects on the child. It may also be the case that the practitioner, as a trusted professional seen regularly by the parent, may hear about their ongoing difficulties. Despite this not being a part of a practitioner's job responsibilities, any support and advice given will not only support the parents, but indirectly be supporting the child.

Illustrative example 2.1

A mother has recently separated from her husband, who was also the father of their two young children. She does not know where he has moved to and is not receiving any financial support from him. As she does not work herself she is in desperate need of money for food and bills. She does not have a telephone or a car and manages the two children in a double buggy.

The mother shares this personal information with the practitioner and asks if they can help. By telephoning the social services department and social security office the practitioner can act as a facilitator to put the mother in contact with the relevant supporting agencies. The mother can take over the telephone once the switchboards have been mastered and the call has been directed to the relevant person.

This one single act could relieve the stress on the mother and thus benefit the children as well. In addition, the setting's awareness of the family situation should lead to appropriate support being offered to the child.

As parents, and therefore 'significant others' in a child's life, parental impact can have considerable effects on the child and also have implications for the setting. Knowledge of a family's culture and value systems is necessary to ensure the appropriateness of tasks offered to the child and of discussions that may occur with all the children attending the setting. As examples, differences may occur in the festivals celebrated by the family, language(s) spoken at home, attitudes to and responses to behaviour, dress, foods and meals. If practitioners do not have knowledge of the relevant cultural beliefs and traditions, then they may inadvertently offend the family or embarrass the child.

A fact as basic as the size of the family can affect children, as only children compared to those with siblings may demonstrate differing abilities to share and take turns, to listen to others and to need more attention than is generally available. A child that is used to having his/her own way and having demands met immediately may find it difficult to settle into the larger group of a setting where the existing children may react quite negatively to such behaviours. The effects of being a part of a step-family, with step-siblings can also affect a young child as their mother may suddenly be sharing her time and attention between more children, and feelings of resentment may arise. Family methods of dealing with behaviours and of behavioural expectations will also vary between families and the routines and rules within the early years setting may be difficult for some children to adapt to on entry. Usually they learn that situational contexts are different and hopefully will respond appropriately and in accordance with the setting's expectations. However, practitioners should be aware of those children who resist the setting's routines and rules, and demonstrate unacceptable behaviours that would otherwise be accepted within their home. Such children will clearly need support and guidance to address any difficulties arising.

It is clear that children can, and will be, affected by a range of family factors. If practitioners accept that children are influenced by their parents and family, then clearly implications arise for reflection. In this era of assessing children holistically we should not overlook factors from inside and outside the setting if we aim fully to assess a child. This will then help to ensure our provision responds directly to the individual needs of the children. Barnes (1995) succinctly summarizes the impact of the family:

> Although other groups and social factors affect socialization, the family is typically seen as the most influential agency in the socialization of the child. It is the context within which the most direct and intimate relationships are forged. Our concept of family is greatly influenced by our personal experiences and our culture. (p. 84)

Families of children with special needs

To discover you are expecting a baby will bring a range of emotions and feelings. Depending on whether the baby was planned or not will clearly have a significant impact and, if unplanned, there may be considerations by the mother and/or the father regarding proceeding with the pregnancy or seeking a termination. Once a mother, with or without the father, accepts to continue with a pregnancy, considerable changes will need to be made for this 'new' future. Hopefully, the news will be greeted with delight and plans will be made to welcome this new life into the family. The impending birth may mean that the mother will have to give up work, either short term or long term, and considerable financial demands will soon become apparent as babies will be costly for many years ahead. Discussions will invariably lead to the child and what he/she may look like, possible names, possible schools and, hopefully, babysitters. Discussions may also explore changes to the life of the family. If the child is the first-born then considerable changes will occur as patterns of socialization will change, along with holidays and trips out. Shopping can become more difficult and the demands on the parents' emotions and feelings will experience changes. Adaptations to the relationship between the parents may be needed to accommodate the emotional and physical demands this important arrival will place on them both. In many cases, it would be hoped that all such considerations will have been made and the required changes will, over time, have been accepted as exciting and positive. To welcome a new baby into any family is generally a time for great celebration.

If problems are detected at routine medical checks during the course of the pregnancy, it may be that parents have to deal with the news that their baby may or will have special needs. The type of need would clearly affect any subsequent decisions and discussions, combined with the family's ability to cope with and provide effectively for the baby. The planned future for their baby, and themselves, will possibly be changed quite dramatically, and all the discussions and family plans that have occurred may need revision. Considerations regarding existing siblings and grandparents may also arise. Should the baby need medical treatment, possibly involving numerous appointments and/or invasive surgery after birth, then implications for time spent in hospital with the baby will arise, combined with the working parent's feelings of not being able to support the family as much due to work commitments. Longer-term plans may also need revisiting. The impact can clearly be considerable for the parents, siblings and extended family members.

At the same time as dealing with the more fundamental practicalities of the news, parents may also be undergoing a range of emotions and feelings that they may, or may not, feel able to share openly. The whole perspective of the family will be affected and at any one time one parent may be undergoing grief at the loss of their planned for child whilst trying to deal with the adaptation to the new child that is on the way. Other emotions experienced could include despair, rejection of the baby, confusion, guilt and/or denial.

Clearly at this difficult time the strength of relationships within the family, both immediate and extended, will play a significant part in the abilities to cope and move forwards. Grandparents, for example, may experience guilt at having children free of difficulties whilst also feeling extremely protective of their own child, the parent-to-be, as parents in general would prefer to carry problems themselves than have their children experiencing them. Conversely, one parent may be coming to terms with the unexpected changes whilst the other is still resistant and finding the situation a considerable strain.

Whether at the pre-natal or post-natal stage, the news that a child is experiencing special needs will have a tremendous impact on the family and as a family, they will need to have ongoing and consistent strengths to cope with the future.

The time of initial diagnosis will require considerable sensitivity from professionals who must be prepared to deal with initial reactions that may vary from parent to parent. Disbelief is a common reaction resulting in the very natural 'Are you sure?' question. Parents may also immediately want answers to a range of diverse questions about the future, and professionals should be able to respond appropriately to all questions that arise. The diagnosis can be made easier or more difficult by the professionals involved, and there exists a plethora of reports of inappropriate professional responses at this time. Professionals dealing with such delicate situations should therefore be suitably qualified and trained in an attempt to support the parents in a positive manner. Carpenter's work (2000) identified reports of 'professional approaches [that] were insensitive and ill-timed' (p. 135) and clearly such instances need redressing.

At this time professionals should also give due acknowledgement to the individual needs of family members as mothers, fathers, grandparents and siblings may each react very differently and require individual attention and consideration. Herbert and Carpenter (1994) reported on the father's 'marginalization' from the situation as they were often expected to be the supportive carer and partner to the mother, which clearly denied them from experiencing their own emotions, feelings and concerns. They concluded that:

> The father's needs were not addressed or, perhaps even noticed. They were seen as the 'supporters' and as such adopted the role society expects – that of being competent in a crisis ... All seven fathers talked of returning to work and trying to search for normality and keep a sense of reality in their lives. (Herbert and Carpenter, 1994, p.27)

If professionals can begin to be aware of the range of difficulties that family members may be experiencing then perhaps the inappropriate handling of situations can be improved in the future. Families who were undergoing difficulties or stresses prior to the diagnosis may be less well placed to deal effectively with this considerable added pressure.

Other special needs may occur or be identified at a later stage. Whilst similar issues for family members are likely to arise, the fact that a child may have been developing according to expected developmental guidelines and has suddenly or gradually deteriorated, will also mean the parents experience a sense of 'losing' their child and finding they are now dealing with a significantly different child. This different situation may well give rise to new challenges and issues relating to both the practical and emotional needs of family members. This would most likely be the case if a child is suggested to have, or is later diagnosed with, autism.

Families of children with autism

For parents of children with autism the same difficulties and feelings would be likely to arise as those discussed in the preceding section, but if diagnosis follows a period of apparent 'normal' development, then the difficulties and issues can be compounded. Again, family structure will have an impact on abilities to cope, combined with the strength of the family prior to diagnosis. Clearly, a single parent will need to bear the responsibilities and stresses single-handed without a partner's support. The considerable demands of a child with autism will create pressures for the single parent who may already be coping with being the only source of practical and emotional support to other siblings. Parenting in general is demanding, but for single parents these demands are multiplied many times over.

Accounts from parents of children with autism are plentiful and give readers, and in particular practitioners, a very real insight into the difficulties they have faced and continue to face. These difficulties are often compounded by the confusion arising from seeing a diverse range of professionals and having to fit in an array of appointments on a fairly consistent and regular basis. Bill Davis, one such parent, stated that despite the local doctor being inconclusive about his son's difficulties and regression, he did not see a need to refer the family further. Davis (2001) continues: 'So we set out on our burdensome journey of psychiatrist, neurologists, MRIs and hearing tests. We scheduled things very quickly, but it still took a few months to follow through with all the appointments' (p. 35). With his wife, Bill had researched widely, and together they were convinced that their son was demonstrating classic autistic behaviours; they simply wanted confirmation. This, they hoped, would enable access to appropriate treatment and educational programmes, and give them the support and direction they wanted and needed. However, it was an ongoing struggle that was compounded by the fact that many specialists appeared reluctant to use the term 'autism'.

Throughout the stages of their child's regression parents may be confused with what is happening and simply unable to make sense of it. If it is their first child and they do not have contact with young children they may initially consider this time as fairly standard for young children. Some will seek information from any available source, the health centre, library, bookshops, friends and/or the Internet, but until a time of diagnosis arrives there will most likely be uncertainty with an underlying knowledge that something is just not right. Not all parents will see a need to seek information but will just wait until such time as a professional raises concerns. Such parents, even when it has been suggested that their child may have autism, may not desire to research information. This is not to say they are any less interested; they are just happy to wait until professionals refer them or suggest ideas for them to follow up. It is probably fair to say, however, that the majority of parents seeing this gradual, yet significant, regression in their child have a strong drive to find out information to ensure they offer the best opportunities to their child.

As previously discussed autistic spectrum disorders comprise three key areas of difficulty: social interaction, social communication and imagination (the triad of impairments). Allied difficulties of repetitive behaviours are also likely to occur. As family interactions are so crucial to the well-being of any family, the effects of a child with autism are likely to have a major impact on the family dynamics. The stresses of caring for a child with autism may leave a parent with little time or energy for either his/her partner and/or other children. Trying to manage a house full-time, undertaking school runs and shopping are all demanding tasks, but for the parent of a child with autism this will be magnified. Families therefore have to be strong before the child with autism can be accommodated with the least effect on individual family members.

The child with autism will appear aloof and withdrawn, may not have a desire to interact with other family members, may be content to line up cars for long periods of time, demonstrate unacceptable or inappropriate behaviours, rock, sway or flap their hands and be resistant to new activities or changes to routines. For children who have previously appeared to be developing along accepted developmental paths there will be a loss of physical contact and two-way interaction. So much so, that the parent may feel that nothing is given back from the child, which is always difficult to deal with as a parent, but even more so if previously such interactions were commonplace. Hugs, kisses and a shared storytime may no longer occur. The child with autism may have little or no sense of danger and may need supervision for much of the day for reasons of safety. Within the family home this can create immense difficulties and resentment amongst some family members.

Trips outside of the home, even to the supermarket, can become traumatic as the child will need attention and may resist holding hands or sitting in a supermarket trolley. Unfortunately, such experiences can be further compounded by lack of public awareness and understanding. Members of the public are likely to stare or avoid the family and may make unhelpful and hurtful comments, often assuming the child is being naughty and the parent is incapable of controlling them. Such attitudes can have significant effects on all family members and, whilst it is hoped that as a society we are moving towards greater acceptance of difference, there are still many who will find this difficult. If this is further exacerbated by the child screaming or hand-flapping and rocking, members of the public can react negatively, through their ignorance. Parents may choose to avoid such trips by leaving one adult at home with the child whilst the rest of the family go out. Brothers and sisters may feel embarrassed and uncomfortable and not wish to go out, whilst others may develop mature levels of understanding, support and protective qualities towards not only their sibling, but also the parent who is bearing the brunt of the problems. Whatever the outcome, it is likely that all family members will be significantly affected.

Shared family shopping trips, perhaps with lunch out, are valuable occasions for all families, so to be in a position where this opportunity is denied your family can lead to resentment. Conversely, it could be argued that the siblings and parents benefit from the 'normality' of such occasions when the child with autism stays at home, as they will have uninterrupted time and attention from the adult with them.

CASE STUDY 2.1

Oliver was referred to a local special needs unit at the age of 2 years and 6 months. He was the youngest of three children born to his parents, Mike and Sue, who lived in the family home in a rural village. Oliver's mother and the health visitor were both concerned about his development and he had recently been referred for a full developmental assessment with the consultant paediatrician.

Oliver had been politely asked to leave his local day nursery due to his complex and often inappropriate behaviours. Despite their best efforts the staff has been unsuccessful in providing for Oliver's needs or securing specialist support and advice. Due to the concerns of many other parents Mike and Sue were asked to withdraw Oliver.

Within the activity room of the special needs unit Oliver appeared fascinated by doors and, in particular, hinges, which he liked to lick. On entry to the room he would run to the home corner and kneel on the floor opening and shutting all the doors repeatedly and only pausing to lick the hinges and catches. Oliver would walk away if anyone approached him or spoke to him, preferring to decline any interaction either verbal or social.

If his name was called he would place his hands over his eyes (not his ears), scream and stamp his feet repeatedly. Oliver ignored both the people and the activities taking place and would not participate in circle time, storytime or snack time. Oliver's mother, Sue, spent considerable periods of time talking to the head of the unit and it was evident that she lacked support and was concerned for Oliver, the rest of the family and the future. She had slept little since Oliver was born and despite initial periods of usual progress, including some speech, interaction and play, the quite sudden regression and subsequent difficulties were having an enormous impact on the family. Sue had been asked by the local post office and stores not to take Oliver in any more as other shoppers, all local villagers, had complained and on several occasions he had bitten other children or adults. As this was the only local shop this clearly created a problem. Sue had begun taking Oliver to the local mother and toddler group but again had received unwelcome comments and felt unable to pursue this venture. Even the local school asked Sue not to take Oliver to open assemblies and concerts as he was too disruptive. Her local friends had slowly withdrawn their friendship and ceased inviting her, Oliver and his siblings for afternoon play sessions.

Sue and Oliver had become more and more isolated. In addition Sue's relationship with her husband had deteriorated as the pressures of caring for Oliver took precedence over most other family and relationship issues. Mike resented the lack of time with Sue and the general problems of living with a young child with autism that did not respond to him in any way. He was in denial about the severity of Oliver's difficulties and was certain that once he started mainstream school everything would 'slot into place'.

▶

▶

> Sue had a feeling that Oliver might be autistic but neither the family doctor nor health visitor would confirm this. She was optimistic about the impending assessment by the consultant paediatrician and hoped that this would result in a diagnosis and intervention support. She was adamant that with a diagnosis she could then state clearly to people that he was not a naughty child but could not help his behaviour.
>
> Sue clearly acknowledged the extent of Oliver's difficulties and was coping admirably under the circumstances, but the impact on her and the rest of the family was considerable, long term and stressful.

Case study 2.1, albeit lengthy, strives to enhance the understanding of autism by making it 'real'. This scenario was of a real family whom I met many years ago, with Oliver being one of the first children with more severe autism than I had ever encountered at that time. Summarizing the key issues will hopefully highlight to practitioners the effects on, and needs of, the members of this family and many others like them:

- relationship difficulties between husband and wife;

- exclusion from the local shop, school events and mother and toddler group;

- lack of local friendships offering social contact for the parents and/or the family as a whole unit;

- the mother's perceived need for a diagnosis;

- the father's denial and belief that all will be well following school entry;

- the mother's need to talk to another adult about her son and the difficulties the family was experiencing;

- the lack of local supporting networks;

- difficulties incurred by Oliver's siblings;

- practical and emotional stresses of coping from day to day;

- the need for accessible information.

After a period of initial assessment in the unit, by the staff and the visiting speech and language therapist, Oliver was given a key worker who devoted considerable amounts of time to establishing a relationship with him. Over the subsequent three years he remained at the unit and made slow but steady progress in all areas. With the use of Makaton (see Chapter 5) he was enabled to begin communication and he would allow his key worker to play and work directly with him, and other adults and children to play near him. He participated in social activities as far as he was able, by sitting as a part of the group, although not interacting with the activities. Sue was initially heavily supported by the staff and continued to need time to talk on a regular basis. Other systems had been put in place following a diagnosis of autism at the age of 3 years 11 months, which included respite care once a month for a whole day. This enabled the family to re-establish more usual family activities. Oliver's difficulties did not disappear but, with appropriate intervention and a network of multidisciplinary working, Sue become empowered to help her son's progress in a positive way and to reduce her isolation. Oliver's difficulties would also change as he matured, as with all children, but with continued support it was hoped that progress would be consistent and the limiting effects of autism would be reduced through the effective use of appropriate strategies working within Oliver's world and utilizing his strengths and abilities. The provision enabled him to participate more fully in the world around him. Practitioners need to appreciate and understand the effects of autism on the child but also to reflect on the needs of the family members to ensure effective support for them is in place.

To further develop our understanding of the needs of individual family members, parents, siblings and grandparents will be considered independently, but this should not detract the reader from the interrelationships that coexist.

Parents of children with autism

Some of the key difficulties experienced by parents have already been discussed, but expansion and clarification is now pertinent. All adults will have their own understanding of disability and some may have knowledge or experience of children with autism, but in addition to this knowledge they will have knowledge about their relationship with their partner and other family members. Their reactions to a diagnosis of autism will therefore be affected by their emotional attachment to the child. Their perspectives on disability may be somewhat altered by the personal nature of the scenario and may differ from the views of the professionals they meet, having the additional strong, emotional bond. When this is combined with the loss of a child that appeared to be developing according to standard norms, parental emotions may be further heightened. The feelings of loss, grief, guilt, injustice and despair already identified will have a significant effect on their ability to take on board additional news and information which will clearly have a significant impact on their own future and that of their family.

It may be that a diagnostic assessment is undertaken and the findings are conveyed at a meeting at which only one of the parents can attend due to family or work commitments. The other parent will therefore be hearing this important information second-hand and possibly lacking some of the detail. In addition, some important questions may arise outside the meeting that can no longer receive an immediate response from the diagnosing professional. Parents' abilities to deal with a diagnosis of autism will vary from individual to individual, but a range of emotions, feelings and concerns will be likely to emerge as they try to assimilate the information that will clearly have a long-term and significant impact on their family. This time of diagnosis is therefore crucial and support may well be needed. Some parents may need to go away to think and talk, and then come back at a later date to resume the discussion with the professional.

Research has shown that the time and nature of the diagnosis is still an area needing improvement as parents are often dissatisfied with their own experiences. Dale (1996) comments that:

> Parents complain about delays and evasion in the telling, being given false assurances, being told in an abrupt and uncaring way, having the negative consequences of the child's condition emphasized, each parent being told separately, being left to break the news to the other parent, being told in a public place, and not being given access to a private place afterwards. (p. 51)

Problems also exist around securing the diagnosis in the first place. In some areas of the country a consultant paediatrician will undertake this, while in other areas it may be a clinical psychologist or even an autism specific developmental assessment unit. Due to this variance there is an issue of equality of access for all parents regardless of where they live. Again, many parents have reported on their struggles to secure diagnoses, such as Lady Astor (Internet 6), who first took her daughter Olivia to a paediatrician at age 19 months. This resulted in the suggestion that Olivia was a 'late developer'. A later hospital visit resulted in a diagnosis that Olivia had 'special needs' and a subsequent visit to a child development professional added little to the puzzle, although by this time Lady Astor had realized that Olivia's behaviours were classically autistic. At this time Lady Astor embarked on a regime of alternative therapies in her attempt to try to help her daughter overcome her difficulties. It was only when she was offered a National Autistic Society leaflet that she firmly believed that she was dealing with a child with autism, for which a diagnosis followed when Olivia was 5 years old.

Clearly such stories indicate the difficulties some parents can experience whilst trying to clarify their understanding of their child's difficulties. When delays and unhelpful diagnoses are offered this simply compounds the parents' overall stresses and concerns, especially when we consider the routine day-to-day management difficulties they are already undergoing within the family.

Due to the complex nature of autistic spectrum disorders, children with this disorder will naturally demand the majority of the parents' time on a daily basis. This may result in the other children of the family feeling left out and resentful. Quality time with any other child in the family may be severely restricted by the need to keep attending to the needs of the child with autism during this 'special time'. The sibling may then feel deprived of the parent's full attention which, over a prolonged period of time, can have significant effects. Whilst they may, if mature enough, understand the need for the parent to attend to the child with autism, a natural resentment and jealousy may occur. If the parents are working on particular positive reinforcement strategies with the child with autism, they will be constantly rewarding the child verbally or non-verbally. This could result in siblings feeling that they cannot command such frequent and regular positive responses and thus could perceive their achievements to be less important. Despite their love for all their children the parents may be unaware of these feelings in their other children and may not therefore be able to respond appropriately to redress this imbalance. This has implications for all practitioners, whether they are providing for a child with autism, or a sibling of a child with autism, as the resulting effect could be lowered self-esteem and lack of desire to continue trying to succeed. Their motivation could be severely compounded.

Parents ideally need a reliable and trustworthy babysitter who is familiar with their child and the child with them. It is common to assume that no one else can cope with your child, but time for the parents to be together and also for the parents to participate in activities with the other siblings is essential to maintain a level of ordinary family life. The benefits of such a babysitter would be many, but predominantly would offer respite and a welcome breathing space for family members.

One of the major concerns for parents of children with autism is the future and what will happen. After receiving a diagnosis questions will frequently arise: 'what happens next?' and 'what will happen in the future for the child with autism and other family members?' Concerns relate to future educational opportunities, the possibility of employment and independent living, public reactions when out of the home undertaking 'normal activities', how to deal with issues of sexuality, the list goes on. Adults with autism may well demonstrate unusual or inappropriate behaviours which, due to their adult size, are more pronounced. I know an adult who when walking along the street will take six paces forwards, crouch down to the ground, spring up and clap his hands. For him there is nothing unusual about this as he is unable to comprehend that it is not accepted behaviour when in public and is likely to achieve many negative comments and stares. It is probably more difficult for the carer he is with.

Siblings of children with autism

Possibly the most important issue for siblings is the need for information at every stage of their lives, to enable their understanding of what is going on, what is likely to happen next and why. Clearly this will need to be in age-appropriate language to enable understanding. For young children, books such as *My Brother is Different* by Louise Gorrod (1997) and *Children with Autism: A Booklet for Brothers and Sisters* by Julie Davies (n.d.), are two excellent examples of useful texts in storybook form with clear pictures which can be very helpful when shared with other young children. These could be used with siblings in the home, children of friends, children within the extended family, but also within an early years setting. As we are all aware, young children love to share a storybook with an adult, and such a book, whilst having a poignant meaning, is simply an enjoyable storybook to most young children. The National Autistic Society is a useful source of such texts for siblings of all ages (Internet 7, publications pages). If storybooks and texts are used in conjunction with regular opportunities to talk openly about issues, then the family will be setting up an appropriate forum in which to deal with the siblings' issues. Children should realize early on that they are entitled to their own feelings and emotions, and to share them with those around is valuable, helping to ensure understanding of their perspective. Siblings will need time to feel valued and loved equally, and time to talk, be respected and communicate. Opportunities to meet with other siblings of children with autism could be particularly helpful as they will share many common issues and concerns. It is also very helpful and supportive to discover there are others in the same position as them.

Sibling relationships for all children would normally begin to develop before or from birth. Around the ages of 3 or 4, younger siblings will be at a stage of development which supports playing with their siblings in an appropriate way and this time is one of great bonding for them. We are all aware that siblings will fight, squabble and argue, but underneath a strong relationship will be developing. As young children develop into teenagers and young adults the form of this relationship will change, often resulting in a period of not getting along with a teenage sibling, but, generally speaking, the earlier closeness will return in adulthood. If a sibling has autism then he/she will not have a need to establish such a relationship with you or anyone, and siblings may find this difficult to deal with and accept. Again talking about the situation would be helpful at this juncture.

One key area of difficulty is that of the sibling with autism spoiling or interfering with the activities of their siblings. They may enter a child's bedroom and dismantle the brick castle that is in mid-construction, enjoying the sound the bricks make when they crash onto the floor. Unable to understand their sibling's feelings and anger at this, they may laugh when the sibling begins shouting at them, which could exacerbate the situation further. As a result of such an outburst the child may then be admonished for shouting at their sibling with autism, whilst the sibling is taken with the parent and given a drink. The messages this would give to the child are significant and may have an impact on how they deal with similar situations in the future. There is a need, therefore, for siblings to have their own space where they can be alone, or with family or friends, or be involved in their own activities. Bedrooms are ideal for this purpose but there may be a need for some sort of lock to ensure privacy and the uninterrupted completion of activities. The only potential difficulty with this situation is that siblings may use this 'escape' too much and become isolated themselves.

In addition, siblings may be embarrassed about the behaviour of the child with autism and about public reaction, resulting in them not inviting their own friends to play and not wanting to go out of the house. Yet in many cases siblings will be able to support and help the child with autism make steady progress, by giving them time, showing them how to do things and supporting any specific intervention strategies the family may be using. This in turn could give them a sense of achievement and satisfaction in the knowledge that they are helping their brother/sister and their parents.

Other aspects of having a sibling with autism, or any special need, can also be beneficial to brothers and sisters. Despite difficulties experienced whilst growing up, adults report later that the experience overall gave them increased sensitivity and a sense of responsibility, combined with an awareness of the difficulties experienced by their sibling and a sense of immense pride in their achievements. Their heightened awareness of disability issues and the problems families face will be likely to result in well-informed adults who are not only open to difference, but also are eager to celebrate difference. Generally speaking, they will grow into excellent advocates for disability issues.

In summary, siblings will develop their own feelings about autism, their own knowledge and awareness of autistic issues and their own needs. Practitioners should always be sensitive to issues relating to siblings in order to support any such children in the setting. If you are working with a child who has a sibling with autism your own understanding and awareness of the issues relating to autism and the effects on families will enable you to support them positively.

Grandparents

Grandparents historically tend to be quite heavily involved with their grandchildren. Although family structures have changed over the years and more families live further away from grandparents, the emotional bonds and desire to support will still exist. Even if it is only by way of being on the end of the telephone or email, grandparents can play an important supporting role. As practitioners we may work with grandparents who are taking responsibility for the daily care of their grandchildren and therefore we may see them regularly, but the parents infrequently. It is important that we consider issues directly relating to their own needs as well as their needs as caregivers to their grandchildren. At the same time, however, we should respect the family relationships as not all grandparents have the same views as their own children and it is not always the case that healthy and supportive relationships exist.

When autism is first noticed or diagnosed it may be that the parents inadvertently wish to protect their own parents from the news, but in most cases the grandparents would want to know and be able to offer support in any way they are able. At this difficult time grandparents may have feelings of guilt that they themselves had healthy children, free of difficulties, and would wish to remove the problems from their adult children. They may also experience grief, anger, sorrow and concern at the diagnosis of autism and will need time and support to come to terms with the situation. Their own outdated views of disability and lack of knowledge and understanding of autism could compound the situation further.

If grandparents feel unable to support the child in a practical, hands-on way, then they can still offer great support through alternative means such as finding out information, taking siblings out, taking siblings to school or early years settings, combined with the more practical tasks of shopping, washing and ironing. Some grandparents may feel unable directly to support the child through their own lack of knowledge and awareness and 'fear' of this strange disorder. They may find the behaviours of the child particularly odd or unusual and simply not know how to try to interact or react. With information and support they can learn these things and offer greater support for which they would probably feel a tremendous sense of achievement. Not all grandparents, can offer such specific and specialized help to their grandchildren, which in turn gives them tremendous pleasure and satisfaction. If they feel able to take on responsibilities as respite carers on a regular basis, then family members will be relieved of considerable pressures. It may be that grandparents take time to come to this level of acceptance, but the rewards can be plentiful.

Success or otherwise will greatly depend on the relationships between the parents and grandparents prior to the diagnosis of autism. If grandparents have been heavily and positively involved with their adult children before and after the first grandchild was born, then it is more likely that they will cope better and be more supportive once difficulties emerge. In such a situation, it is likely that discussions will occur regularly, views and feelings will be respected and channels of communication will be open. The care and concern of the grandparents for both their children and grandchild is normally paramount, and grandparents can be excellent at getting involved as and whenever needed to help, which can have tremendous benefits for all family members.

Whether we see grandparents frequently or infrequently we cannot overlook the role they play within any family network, either positively or negatively. Practitioners should therefore be aware of issues pertinent to grandparents in order better to understand the family dynamics and therefore the child. Such issues should be considered within our overall planning and, more importantly, when planning for the individual needs of the child with autism.

Issues for practitioners

To fully support the child with autism practitioners need a good understanding of family related issues. If we see the child as first and foremost, a child within a dynamic family, then we can see that our role is secondary, whilst no less important. To provide appropriately for the child we will need to reflect on all issues affecting them, including their family. We should reflect separately on issues pertinent to mothers, fathers, siblings and grandparents, and acknowledge that we have a role in supporting their needs as well, in order to support the child in a holistic manner. Although we may not often see the grandparents it may be that they see the setting as a source of information for themselves. We may see siblings regularly or now and again, but should be informed sufficiently so we can respect and value their role in the support of the child with autism whom we are working with. Practitioners should, at all times, listen to family members in order to support them more appropriately, which again will lead to improved provision for the child. We are not the 'experts' on their child, the family will always take that role, but we can use information given about the child to help build up a complete picture. Being open to communication and information-sharing will be essential for practitioners. Clearly issues relating to parental partnerships and multidisciplinary working will also be crucial and are also requirements of current legislation and guidance for the early years.

Ongoing research will support developments in all the above areas and should be supported. One such report, entitled *Making a Difference: Early Interventions for Children with Autistic Spectrum Disorders*, was recently published by the National Foundation for Educational Research (NfER), being sponsored by the Local Government Association (LGA) (Evans et al. 2001). Relating specifically to parents, the report highlights a parental need for early recognition of their child's difficulties and subsequent provision, which varied considerably across the country, some parents being quite satisfied whilst others remained dissatisfied. The report further recommends that:

> *A key worker with knowledge and expertise in autistic spectrum disorders should be assigned to each family to give advice and information, and enable them to access the right programme of support for themselves and their child. The key worker should facilitate communication between the various professionals involved and the family. (ibid. p.85)*

This clearly has implications for staff training to ensure all settings can offer a professional with 'knowledge and expertise in autistic spectrum disorders' to families, especially in the current climate of increased inclusion.

Summary

If practitioners wish to support the child through individual, effective and appropriate means, then the effects on all family members should be a key cause for consideration. Families have a tremendous impact on the children within them and we cannot assess a child's needs holistically without due consideration of other family members, family relationships and the dynamics of the family. Ensuring we consider the needs of each family member will also ensure we are considering the family as a whole unit and the child with autism that we are providing for. The more knowledge we have, the more informed our provision will be. Practitioners should therefore consider:

- ■ the sensitive nature of the issues we are dealing with;
- ■ the impact individual family members have on the child with autism;

- the dynamic and evolving nature of the family;

- functioning abilities of the family as a whole;

- the individual perspectives of family members;

- the need to support individual family members;

- the existing support networks within and outside of the family;

- the positive and negative effects of family members on the child with autism;

- the fact that the family knows the child best;

- our own assessment processes – to ensure we consider family issues in an holistic assessment of the child's needs;

- current legislation and guidance relating to autism and specifically supporting families of children with special needs;

- our own working practices with professionals from other disciplines and agencies;

- and always remember that, whilst the child must remain the focus of our work, we should not ignore family issues.

As Wall (2003a) suggests:

Throughout our planning, policy-making and practice we must consider and address, to the best of our ability, the needs of each family member. While the child must always be the key focus of our work, family members must always be considered. This will enhance our work with the child and help him/her to work towards achieving his/her full potential. (p.40)

Key issues

- *The impact of a child with autism on parents, siblings and grandparents must be acknowledged and respected.*

- *The need to support family members must be recognized.*

- *Practitioners need to be aware of all local supporting agencies and individual professionals.*

- *Knowledge and experience of autistic spectrum disorders is essential in order to support family members.*

- *Working practices and policies should reflect this aspect of our work.*

Some suggestions for discussion

Item 1

Focus on one child with autism you are currently providing for. Write a list of all family members that impact on the child's life and for each one attempt to identify the issues that may be creating the most significant difficulties for them at the present time. Discuss as a staff to compile an overall list of key issues.

Item 2

For each of the issues identified in item 1 above, consider what support is currently available and by whom. Identify any gaps in support that may need addressing.

Item 3

Explore the knowledge individual members of staff have of all agencies that could support the needs of a child with autism and/or their family. Consider how accessible this information is to family members and look for ways to improve this valuable source of information and make it accessible to all.

📖 Suggested further reading

Carpenter, B. (2000) 'Sustaining the family: meeting the needs of families of children with disabilities', *British Journal of Special Education*, 27(3), pp. 135–43.

Dale, N. (1996) *Working with Families of Children with Special Needs*. London: Routledge, Chapter 3.

National Autistic Society (NAS) (2000). *Experiences of the Whole Family*. London: NAS.

Wall, K. (2003) *Special Needs and Early Years: A Practitioner's Guide*. London: Sage, Chapter 2.

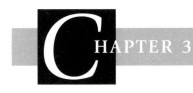

CHAPTER 3

Issues of diagnosis and assessment

Introduction

Having discussed the characteristics and features of autism along with consideration of family issues in the two previous chapters, practitioners will have been alerted to some of the implications for the early years setting and all adults coming into contact with the child. In this chapter issues of diagnosis and assessment will be explored, as early identification, assessment and diagnosis should inform future planning. Practitioners and researchers have often debated the positive and negative aspects of labelling, which could be viewed as an outcome of diagnosis. Whilst labelling may well have a negative impact in some areas, the child with autism will need to be supported by practitioners who have knowledge and understanding of autistic spectrum disorders and how to provide appropriately for children on the autistic spectrum. A diagnosis of autism can therefore be more positive for the child if it will lead to appropriate provision by skilled staff.

The current diagnostic process in the UK can vary according to the professionals involved and the assessments used. This may further vary geographically. Equity of access to meaningful diagnoses will be explored, as will family reactions to the initial diagnosis. The fact that some children will have progressed according to expected development patterns prior to a period of rapid regression would magnify possible feelings of loss. If this is then followed by difficulties securing a diagnosis and a further lengthy period of time before securing a placement, the parents' difficulties would be further compounded.

If practitioners are involved with the child prior to diagnosis then they should be able to contribute valuable information to the diagnostic assessment. Alternatively, it may be practitioners who raise initial concerns about the child which should lead to a diagnostic assessment. The importance of practitioner awareness and understanding of autistic spectrum disorders is once again highlighted as a fundamental element of effective assessment and provision.

Why diagnose?

Siegel (1996) identifies two purposes for diagnosis:

> *First, a diagnosis is a label. It means that what is wrong is a recognizable*
> *problem that has happened before. The 'label' is important in so far as it is a*
> *shorthand for a treatment plan. The second very important purpose of a*
> *'label' or diagnosis is that it is a ticket to services. (p. 82)*

Historically, since the Warnock Report of 1978, we have been moving away from a system that labels children to a system wherein we provide for children's individual needs rather than pigeon-hole them into a category of need or disorder. So it could be suggested that to call for diagnosis, and therefore a label, of an autistic spectrum disorder could be a regressive step. However, within the field of special needs and more specifically considering autistic spectrum disorders, the clarity of a firm diagnosis can be, as Siegel suggested, a clear indication of the type of provision that should follow, assuming practitioner and parental knowledge of the disorder. The danger lies when that knowledge does not exist, as ignorance of the difficulties related to autism could lead to compounding the child's, and thus the family's, difficulties. Opponents of diagnostic processes would argue that expectations could be limited, other difficulties may not be identified and that diagnosis focuses solely on the difficulties within the child. Whilst a successful inclusive education system should be supported, this would depend on a range of issues including practitioner training, access to appropriate training, resources and funding, which currently have not been fully addressed in a comprehensive and nationwide manner. For the child with autism to be placed in a nursery setting where there are no members of staff with adequate knowledge of autism and the implications for the setting, the child's difficulties could be seriously compounded. Therefore, diagnosis should help identify to parents and practitioners alike the implications for all concerned, as well as suggesting appropriate ways forward, to enhance the learning opportunities and thus the future for the child. Although a diagnosis cannot secure appropriate provision, it should inform those involved in the decision-making process. This will further depend on the availability of appropriate provision in each local area.

A key consideration in the debate for and against diagnosis and labelling would be that a diagnosis and subsequent label would, hopefully, inform those working with the child. However, as children with autism can experience behavioural difficulties, language communication difficulties, interaction difficulties, learning difficulties, visual problems and/or hearing problems, a misdiagnosis is possible. If a child presents with severe speech and language difficulties, then these difficulties could overshadow any additional difficulties, and the likely speech and language assessment could exclude consideration of other disorders. If a misdiagnosis of specific language disorder is made the child may be offered a place at a local speech and language unit and, whilst this may support the speech and language difficulties of the child with autism, other difficulties could be ignored. Unless practitioners are aware of the child's autistic difficulties and have a good understanding of autism, they may inadvertently introduce inappropriate strategies. This could result in unusual and severe reactions due to the confusion the child would be experiencing, so a vicious and inappropriate cycle would emerge. Peeters (1997) states convincingly that:

> Their tragedy is that although they are suffering from the developmental
> disorder of autism, they are being treated for mental illness or ordinary mental
> retardation. This is not how it should be, but it is still the case that the quality of
> an autistic person's life depends less on the extent of his handicap and more on
> the place where he was born and whether it is a place where autism is
> properly understood. In this sense diagnostic labels can save lives. (p. 7)

A final issue concerning the need to diagnose relates to those educational authorities who prefer to delay decisions of diagnosing autistic spectrum disorder due to the inferred costs of appropriate provision. Whilst one would think that at the beginning of the twenty-first century we would have progressed beyond such difficulties of funding, they clearly, and sadly, do still exist in some areas. Aarons and Gittens (1999) consider this still to be a major concern:

> It is a fact that in areas where there is no provision, or willingness to finance
> placement in schools elsewhere, autism tends not to exist! It may be given an
> assortment of other labels to accommodate affected children in whatever
> special educational provision is available. Yet in areas where there is
> provision, there is no difficulty filling places. (p. 24)

Some parents may already have an idea that their child is experiencing an autistic spectrum disorder and feel the need for a confirming diagnosis, which is felt will help them to move forwards. Such parents are likely already to have sought out information from friends, professionals, media, the Internet and libraries, and feel confident in their own knowledge of the child and his/her difficulties. Somehow these parents feel that to have a confirmation of the disorder would make life more manageable and offer some direction and security, as the uncertainty will have been removed.

It can be concluded that issues surrounding diagnosis are current and wide-ranging. Debates will continue but we need to be working towards ensuring that any child with autism, wherever they live in the UK, has access to early diagnosis and appropriate intervention.

Delays in the diagnostic process

Any delays in the diagnostic process and subsequent provision will magnify the already existing difficulties of the parents and family of the child with autism. In addition, the two stages of diagnosis and then provision are separated in the UK, with the diagnosing professional's direct involvement (often health authority based) concluding with the writing and distribution of their report. This does not then automatically lead to provision and parents may find themselves working to secure an educational placement through the local education authority. The NAS (1999a) conclude that:

> *The shortage of appropriate educational resources for children with autism takes some parents into an adversarial relationship with their local education authority. You then feel that you have to fight to ensure your child's needs will be met and you realise that this forces you to compete with other parents for scarce resources. (p. 17)*

Jordan, Jones and Murray (1998) undertook research on educational interventions for children with autism and highlighted the gap between diagnosis and provision as a key difficulty for parents. They continued to identify that parents may search themselves for the most appropriate intervention approach but be misinformed by marketing information and claims of guaranteed success, resulting in inappropriate decisions which may prove unsuccessful for their child. Such facts are supported by the NAS research report (1999b) which concluded that:

> *More than 40% of parents had to wait over 3 years to get a diagnosis, 15% had to wait between 5 and 9 years and it took 10% more than 10 years. The mean average time that it took to get a diagnosis was approximately 2 and a half years. (p. 9)*

Clearly issues of access to information, visits to placements, supportive professionals working in a multidisciplinary way and local authority support will be needed to support parents at this difficult and confusing time, but procedural delays should be minimized whenever and wherever possible. Howlin and

Moore's research (1997) into the diagnostic process highlighted that despite nearly half of the parents of the 1,200 children involved identifying problems before the child was 2 years of age, the final diagnosis was not secured until the child was on average, around 6 years of age. This situation was instrumental in the parents' dissatisfaction with the diagnostic experience. Such delays should clearly be avoided.

Difficulties with diagnoses

The research into early interventions undertaken by Evans et al. (2001) indicated general improvement in diagnostic assessments to enable diagnosis in younger children and that training for some professionals had also increased, again supporting the initial diagnosis. However, increased awareness of the characteristics of autism and improved diagnostic systems was creating a concern over possible 'overidentification' or even 'wrong diagnosis'. These will clearly be issues for the future.

Possibly the key difficulty regarding diagnosis is discriminating between autism and other disorders. As outlined in Chapter 1 there are a range of conditions and disorders that result in similar difficulties to those experienced by children with autism, therefore knowledge of, and confidence in, diagnosis will be critical on the part of diagnosing professionals. Aarons and Gittens (1999) suggest that some professionals hold the view that autism is a rare condition, which can affect their diagnoses. Similarly it is not possible to diagnose autism from a blood test, X-ray or scan, as it is the combination of difficulties, peculiar to autism, that inform the diagnosis. Perhaps the ability to eliminate all other conditions would be a worthwhile avenue to reflect on.

The range of pervasive developmental disorders (PDDs) which includes autistic spectrum disorders, also covers Rett's syndrome, PDD-NOS, childhood disintegrative disorder, autism and Asperger's syndrome. Clearly, practitioners need to have a thorough understanding of normal developmental patterns in childhood and the five conditions mentioned above, as well as a clear understanding of all the allied difficulties experienced by children with autism. The knowledge, and therefore the training, of diagnosing professionals is becoming increasingly important to ensure correct diagnoses.

For those children who are considered by health visitors to present with global developmental delay and pronounced speech and language difficulties, the path of referrals may not immediately lead to a professional capable of diagnosing autism. It may be that an initial referral to a speech and language therapist is sought, followed by a referral to the ear, nose and throat department for a full hearing assessment. The results of this could be fed back to the general practitioner (GP) who then refers the family to a paediatrician for a full developmental assessment, the outcome of which could be that the child displays autistic-type tendencies or autistic-type behaviours, so still no secure diagnosis has been achieved. As each referral could incur a wait of several weeks or even months, then the overall timescale can be considerable. If, however, the child is fortunate enough to be seen by a professional early on who is knowledgeable of autistic spectrum disorders, then the whole process leading to a final diagnosis of autism could be quicker, simpler and less stressful for parents. Thus a lottery-type system exists which is clearly inappropriate and raises issues of equity of access to professionals and services for all children with autism wherever they live.

Who diagnoses?

Professionals involved in diagnosing autistic spectrum disorders will vary according to availability of services in each authority. Diagnosing professionals can span health and education departments, but in many cases a combination approach will be used with reports and input from a range of professionals involved with the child, plus information gained from parents. This should culminate in a thorough, detailed and holistic assessment using the knowledge, expertise and experiences of all involved.

Concerns may arise regarding the differing perspectives of professionals diagnosing the disorder and some would suggest that in some areas of the country services are more budget led as opposed to being led by individual children and individual needs. From personal experience I can recall a stage when I was informed by managers that all those working with young children with special needs should refrain from suggesting specific conditions to parents when discussing the children and their needs. Whilst it could be accepted that practitioners should be wary of naming a disorder which subsequently may be proved to be inaccurate, there can be occasions when parents are confident that they know their child's condition and are desperate to receive confirmation. This then enables parents to begin understanding the condition and how they might be able to support their own child. Knowledgeable practitioners, who are respected professionals in their field, should not be restricted in this manner.

The diagnosis of autism is highly specific and requires considerable training and expertise to undertake appropriately, but the final diagnosis should not rest solely with one professional. The range of professionals and parents involved through the process will inform the diagnosing professional and all information should be considered before a diagnosis is made.

Multidisciplinary teams may not be available in some areas and it is here that diagnostic assessments will be crucial to support decisions made by a limited number of professionals. Those involved could include:

■ parents;

■ health visitor;

■ GP;

■ paediatrician or consultant paediatrician;

■ educational psychologist;

■ clinical psychologist;

■ psychiatrist;

■ SENCO;

■ teacher or early years practitioner;

■ social worker;

■ physiotherapist;

■ occupational therapist;

■ speech and language therapist;

■ audiologist;

■ ophthalmologist.

Through careful and skilled interpretation of any reports offered by involved professionals and parents, the whole picture of the child can evolve which should then highlight the child's very individual needs and inform the diagnostic process and future provision.

Which professionals are involved in a diagnostic process will partly depend on what is available locally but also the pathway from initial concerns onwards. As an example, if parents notice difficulties or unexpected changes in their 2-year-old, the first port of call would probably be the local health clinic, GP or health visitor. At this point the professional may suggest monitoring for a while to assess further progress and development, but for others a referral to an outside professional may happen straight away. This could be the speech and language therapist or audiologist, to rule out problems in those areas. This would likely be followed by a referral to a paediatrician or local assessment centre.

The lack of a standard route to diagnosis can be very confusing for parents. After raising initial concerns with the health visitor the parents may feel uncertainty and concern for the outcomes, and to be suddenly faced with a confusing range of appointments with professionals they did not consider they would need to meet can be daunting. Terminology, jargon and reports can be disempowering to parents who previously felt in control of their own lives and parenting abilities. Careful handling of any such referrals should therefore be a consideration for involved professionals and was a recommendation in the report by Evans et al. (2001). The NAS report (1999b) concluded that of 268 families reviewed 65 per cent saw three or more professionals prior to diagnosis and 23 per cent saw five or more. The report states that: 'This is another reason why so much time is wasted in the struggle to get a diagnosis. Parents also mentioned in their general comments that they felt professionals often left them in the dark – sometimes deliberately' (Ibid., p. 13). The latter part of the quote refers to the reluctance to diagnose autism due to the lack of appropriate resources and provision to cater for the child's needs, which was highlighted earlier in this chapter.

Components of a diagnostic assessment

Historically, diagnostic assessments of young children with autism have varied, depending on a range of factors including diagnostic test used, local availability of diagnosing professionals and the range of professionals undertaking the diagnoses. This raised many issues including the question of validity. Over the past 20 years the whole process has become more standardized, as indicated by a recent Medical Research Council (MRC) review stating: 'Recently, systematic assessment tools for history taking and observation have been developed, lessening the reliance on clinical judgement' (Internet 9). The triad of impairments is, however, reflected in most of the current assessment schedules.

The more recently developed assessment tools such as the Revised Autism Diagnostic Interview (ADI), the Autism Diagnostic Observational Schedule (ADOS) and the Diagnostic Interview for Social and Communication Disorders (DISCO) each allow the collation of data from a range of sources by a well-trained professional with extensive knowledge and experience of autistic spectrum disorders. It would therefore be inappropriate for early years practitioners to diagnose autism without being part of a full assessment and diagnostic team.

Since the 1970s, much debating has taken place regarding the most effective basis for clinical diagnosis and a range of options has been considered.

Consideration of all these areas would be recommended:

- Past history of child:

    - information from parents (which will partly depend on accuracy of recall),

    - observations from home and early years setting,

    - information gathered from professional reports,

    - evidence of child's 'work' (drawings etc.),

    - results of prior professional testing;

- current observations made by the diagnosing professional;

- results of autism specific diagnostic assessments;

- collation of information from all the above.

As previously stated, such diagnoses should only be undertaken by experienced professionals with a wealth of knowledge and skills in autistic spectrum disorders combined with training in the use of the chosen diagnostic assessment.

Screening instruments which can be used with children under the age of school entry have also been developed to give an indication of autistic spectrum disorders. The reliability of such screening systems is still subject to ongoing research as they tend to be fairly brief and thus lacking in detail. The two main screening tools are:

1. *Checklist for Autism in Toddlers (CHAT) for use with children aged 18–42 months.* Devised by Baron-Cohen et al. in 1992, the CHAT aims to indicate the likelihood of a later diagnosis of autism. Concerns at the time about the lack of diagnoses during the first five years of life, the lack of knowledge and skills of diagnosing professionals and the difficulties identifying autism, as opposed to allied difficulties, prompted the research programme which culminated in the CHAT screening test. It was felt by the team that earlier diagnoses would be beneficial to both the children and their families as it should result in earlier and appropriate interventions to be set in place. Comprising two sections, the first is completed by the child's parents and the latter by the health visitor, with both sections focusing on joint attention and pretend play. Section one asks specific questions of the parent requiring only Yes or

No answers and the professional's section involves setting up five simple pretend play situations and observing, noting and commenting on the child's reactions. An example is using a child-sized teapot and cup and asking the child to make a cup of tea, which most children of 18 months would be able to interpret, demonstrate and enjoy, but would be difficult for a young child with autism. The scoring of the test is very simple with several key questions indicating the possibility of later diagnosis of autism. In this case the child would be monitored at regular intervals.

2. *Childhood Autism Rating Scale (CARS) for children aged 24 months+*. Devised by Reichler and Schopler in 1971 the CARS was later published in 1980 (Schopler et al., 1980). Schopler, Reichler and Renner (1986) state that: 'the CARS is a 15-item behavioural rating scale developed to identify children with autism. It further distinguishes children with autism in the mild and moderate range from children with autism in the moderate to severe range' (p. 1). The CARS is a straightforward and simple checklist which can be filled in by a professional who knows the child well. The 15 items listed cover areas such as relating to people, body use and adaptation to change, and each item contains four written statements. A circle is placed around the number of the statement which describes the child most accurately. There is also a space for any observational comments in each section. The total of scores is then calculated with scores between 30 and 60 indicating autism. The screening test was standardized on the performances of over 1,500 children. Being simple to use the CARS could be used to confirm concerns that a child *might* be on the autistic spectrum prior to a multidisciplinary diagnostic assessment but also supports individual planning for the child. Whilst not intended to be used as a detailed diagnostic tool, the CARS is a useful indicator, as supported by the NAS: 'It [the CARS] also distinguishes the degree of autism. It takes about 30–45 minutes to administer and is widely regarded as a reliable tool for diagnosing autism' (Internet 10).

Diagnostic instruments

Whilst the CHAT and CARS are screening tools to indicate the likelihood of autism, diagnostic assessment tools are more detailed and thorough assessments that would be undertaken by trained and experienced professionals such as consultant paediatricians, clinical psychologists or autism specific assessment teams. Ideally these should be a key feature of a much wider, multidisciplinary assessment process taking into account the medical background, developmental background, current reports, other assessments that have been undertaken plus parental views. The two most well-known, and world-renowned, diagnostic tools are the International Classification of Diseases (ICD-10) developed for the World Health Organization (WHO, 1993), and the Diagnostic and Statistical Manual version four (DSM-lV) developed by the American Psychiatric Association in 1994. Both are only generally administered by psychiatric professionals and can be summarized as follows:

The ICD-10: based on the areas of social interaction, social communication and stereotypical, ritualistic and repetitive behaviours (including resistance to change), the assessments cover the triad of impairments. In addition, the ICD-10 demands that all other possible conditions and disorders have been ruled out. Within each of the three sections relating to the triad of impairments there are five statements, of which the child must demonstrate at least three to warrant a diagnosis of autism.

The DSM-lV comprises three sections. The first then separates further to include the three areas of the triad of impairments, the second looks at onset prior to the age of 3 years plus abnormal levels of function in social interaction, communication and imaginative play, with the third section eliminating the possibility of Rett's syndrome or childhood disintegrative disorder.

Other diagnostic assessments would include (in alphabetical order):

■ Autism Behaviour Checklist – ABC (Krug, Arick and Almond, 1980). The ABC focuses on the detailed behaviours of the child in such areas as language, social, sensory, use of body and objects.

■ Autism Diagnostic Interview – ADI (Le Couter et al., 1989; Rutter et al., 1988). A highly structured and detailed parent interview which can take over an hour, and often considerably longer, to administer. The interview focuses on the areas of communication, social development (including interaction), play and imagination, and behaviours, and provides in-depth detail of the child's development. The ADI is deemed highly reliable.

■ Autism Diagnostic Observation Schedule – ADOS (Lord et al., 1989). The ADOS is based on a developmental approach aiming to distinguish between autism and normal development or mental handicap, and offers an observational assessment of the child. Using specific activities the child would be assessed in the areas within the triad of impairments.

- Behaviour Observation Scale for Autism – BOS (Freeman et al., 1978; Freeman, Ritvo and Schroth, 1984). Using video-taped observations the BOS enables the coding of behaviours when reviewing the tape.

- Behavioural Summarized Evaluation – BSE (Barthélémy et al., 1992). Specifically focuses on the behaviour difficulties demonstrated by children with autism.

- Diagnostic Checklist for Behaviour-Disturbed Children – E2 (Rimland, 1971). Based on Kanner's original definitions of autism, this parent checklist would be completed by the professional and aims to confirm a diagnosis of early infantile autism.

- Diagnostic Interview for Social and Communication Disorders – DISCO (originally the Handicaps and Behaviour Schedule – HIBS: Wing and Gould, 1978). The DISCO was developed to specifically explore areas of child behaviour from infancy upwards, to indicate that a child lies on the autistic spectrum.

- Infant Behavioural Summarized Evaluation – IBSE (Adrien et al., 1992). This adaptation of the BSE supports identification in younger children from 6 months to 4 years,

- Pre-Linguistic Autism Diagnostic Observation Schedule – PL-ADOS (DiLavore, Lord and Rutter, 1995). The PL-ADOS uses a free-play based approach to observe the child's behaviour in areas such as imagination, resistance to change, separation from parent and attention.

Components of diagnosis

Whilst the above diagnostic tools are extremely useful, they should only form a part of the overall diagnosis process, as previously highlighted. When added to the additional observations and reports from parents and professionals involved with the child, a clearer picture should emerge which will inform the diagnosis. However, the collation of such a range of reports, including speech and language reports, audiology reports, diagnostic assessments and parental and practitioner reports, will clearly take time if the diagnostic process is to

explore all supporting information and include full and detailed consideration of all influencing factors whilst also ruling out other conditions.
Although parents may desire a more rapid response, the process should not be
rushed unduly as a diagnosis, or worse a misdiagnosis, will have long-term
consequences. The outcome of a thorough and effective diagnosis should clarify issues to parents and inform future plans for both parents and early years
settings. It should always be remembered that there is no single quick, simple
test to diagnose autistic spectrum disorders, and for diagnoses to be meaningful
they need to be thorough and undertaken by a range of professionals as well as
involving the parents and the child, if he/she is able to make an input. Baron-
Cohen and Bolton (1993) echo the need for full and thorough assessments:

> But the clinic based assessment is only part of the whole assessment. If
> necessary, the picture is further built up by observing the child at home and
> at the school or nursery, during play, and in situations in which natural
> communication and social interaction should be occurring … This process is
> lengthy simply because autism can be confused with other conditions. (p. 15)

It could also be argued that effective provision should not necessarily depend
on a diagnosis of autism. Effective provision for a child with special needs,
including those with autism or suspected as having autism, should involve
play based observations and assessment as part of the ongoing working practices of the setting. Combined with regular interaction with the child's parents
this will identify the child's strengths, weaknesses, areas of difficulty, likes, dislikes and learning styles. From this point, appropriate planning can take place
to incorporate provision directly responding to the individual child's needs.
This perspective is supported by the recent government guidance document
on providing for children with autistic spectrum disorders (ASDs):

> It is important that a child's individual needs are identified as soon as possible
> so that they can be met in the most appropriate way. Assessment over time may
> indicate an ASD but early intervention appropriate to a child's identified needs
> should not be dependent on diagnosis of an ASD. However, a diagnosis may
> help to guide families and professionals to the most appropriate sources of
> information and support networks. (DfES/DoH, 2002, pp. 16)

After the diagnosis

Following the verbal feedback from the diagnosing professional a written
report will usually follow which should be sent to parents and all involved

professionals. The times of initial feedback, and the subsequent content of the report, are very sensitive as the parents may still be trying to come to terms with the diagnosis and implications, as discussed in Chapter 2. The verbal feedback should be delivered by an appropriate professional who can answer at least the majority of questions the parents need immediate answers to, and be knowledgeable as to the likely next steps for the child and the family. Knowledge of appropriate supporting networks will also be essential. Whilst professionals should not give false or unrealistic expectations and hopes to parents, they should be sure to paint a positive picture overall, even if the parents do not feel particularly positive at that point in time.

The report itself should be specific and succinct with minimal jargon and professional terminology, which may confuse parents, make them feel distanced from the process and inferior. Whilst everyone needs to be aware of the difficulties the child is currently experiencing, there should be a balance between strengths as well as weaknesses. The fact that parents may have experienced a range of unexpected appointments, tests and assessments with their child, can, if professionals are not sensitive, make the parents feel a sense of losing control. All professionals involved should use the same terminology when discussing the child, as terms such as autistic-type behaviours, autistic traits or severe language and communication disorder, when related to the same child, can only confuse parents even further. Clarity is therefore essential. Sadly, the NAS report (1999b) on issues of diagnosis found that: 'Not surprisingly, 43% of parents were dissatisfied to some degree with the diagnostic process with 22% being very dissatisfied. In addition, 52% of those parents who were given no assessment of severity were dissatisfied to some degree' (p. 18).

Clearly the outcomes of diagnoses are very sensitive for professionals and parents alike, but with knowledge, expertise and sensitivity, it would be hoped that some of the negative reports from past experiences of the diagnostic process will remain in the past and that improvements will be forthcoming. Building on the extensive research evidence, much progress can be made which would be beneficial to parents and children alike.

Summary

Throughout this chapter a range of issues surrounding diagnosis and assessment have been highlighted and discussed, hopefully clarifying understanding of the diagnostic process. The fact that there can be so many inherent difficulties with a definitive diagnosis will have raised awareness and understanding for parents and professionals. Early identification, diagnosis and early intervention that is tailored to the child's individual needs is imperative if practitioners aim to ensure that young children with autism are given the appropriate support they need to develop skills, which in turn will help them to achieve their full potential. Consideration of the parents' needs and that of the extended family must be seen as a key element of the diagnostic and assessment process.

Practitioners can support the process by undertaking regular observations and assessments of the child they are working with to inform their own planning as well as informing parents and other professionals. Working in an early years setting that regularly interacts with the child and his/her family places practitioners in a position of privileged knowledge and understanding of the family and their needs. The setting will probably be the most frequently used source of support and advice by the parents, so an understanding of the processes and how best to support family members, as well as the child, should be central to the overall provision. Effective collaboration and liaison between all involved professionals will also play a major role in the success, or otherwise, of the diagnostic process. There is no simple test to diagnose autism, but parents and early years practitioners will inform the process considerably, for the good of the child and the family as a whole.

Key issues

- ■ *The diagnostic process is complex, but attention to detail, thoroughness and sensitivity will be needed throughout.*

- ■ *Diagnostic tools are only one part of an holistic diagnostic assessment.*

- ■ *Particular sensitivity of all the issues for families will be needed at the time of diagnosis and immediately following.*

- ■ *Reports should be positive overall, succinct and free of jargon.*

- ■ *Ongoing observations and assessments in early years settings will be fundamental to the diagnostic process as well as informing planning and provision.*

Some suggestions for discussion

Item 1

Consider the possible difficulties faced by parents when a diagnosis of autism is given for their 3-year-old-son. How would your early years setting be able to support them at this time and afterwards?

Item 2

Are all practitioners in your setting familiar with the local pathway to diagnosis for parents from the time of initial concerns onwards? Compile a list or chart signifying to all staff which professionals would be involved in your area and the likely sequence of events?

Item 3

Referring to the pathway created in item 2 above, plan the development of a support pack or information leaflet for parents who will be preparing for the diagnostic process. Consider issues of simplicity, clarity and sensitivity in presentation.

Suggested further reading

Aarons, M. and Gittens, T. (1999) *The Handbook of Autism: A Guide for Parents and Professionals*. 2nd edn. London: Routledge, Chapters 4 and 5.

Howlin, P. (1998) *Children with Autism and Asperger Syndrome. A Guide for Practitioners and Carers*. Chichester: Wiley, Chapter 3.

National Autistic Society (1999) *Diagnosis – Reactions in Families*. London: National Autistic Society.

National Autistic Society (1999) *Opening the Door. A Report on Diagnosis and Assessment of Autism and Asperger Syndrome Based on Personal Experiences*. London: National Autistic Society.

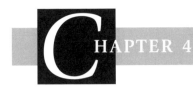

Understanding the world of the child with autism

Introduction

Before we are able to help and support children with autism we, as parents and professionals, need to have a thorough understanding of the world the child is living in, which we will discover is very different from our own. If we cannot begin to explore and understand the ways in which children with autism react to the world around them, then our support may be at best limited, but at worst may inadvertently make their experiences more severe.

When presented with a young child with autism, whether in the home or in an early years setting, we may be presented with a child that has no reason to communicate with us, to play with us, to react to our verbal and non-verbal communication or to accept or even desire any physical contact with us. If a young child falls over and bangs his/her head, then we would generally react by rushing to pick them up, hugging them, drying their tears, comforting them and attempting to calm them down. A young child with autism may make little or no response to the bump on the head and only begin screaming when we pick them up. This unusual response can be disconcerting if we are unfamiliar with children with autism.

To enable increased understanding this chapter will begin to unravel the somewhat different world of the child with autism. Looking at the effects of the triad of impairments and exploring each component separately will help to inform our knowledge and will hopefully support and inform future practice. The area of sensory difficulties will also be considered separately. It may be that the scenarios and short case studies sound familiar to those readers who work with young children with autism, but the supplementary information will hopefully then offer further enlightenment, supporting future progress for the children and the way we work and play with them.

Key areas of difficulty

Reflecting back to the triad of impairments identified in Chapter 1 reminds us of the three key areas of difficulty experienced by children with autism:

- social interaction;

- social communication;

- imagination.

These difficulties are usually accompanied by repetitive and stereotypical behaviours. It should also be remembered that not all children will necessarily experience all the difficulties discussed and those difficulties that are experienced by some, or many, children will vary in their severity from mild to severe. As with all young children, those with autism should be considered as individual children first and foremost who need support in some areas of their development.

The family and their coping strategies should also be considered as they will have a significant impact on the child. The family will have already identified the key areas of difficulty for their own child and will have most likely developed very effective strategies to respond to these. This information will be crucial to the early years practitioner as consistency of approach between home and setting will benefit the child considerably. To introduce separate and contradictory strategies will confuse a child that specifically needs routine and familiarity. For an effective partnership with the parents this two-way sharing of information should be a natural part of our process of provision.

Social interaction

Looking back at the list of eight behaviours relating to social interaction, given in Chapter 1, already gives us a basic understanding of the areas a child with autism may have particular difficulty with. From only a few weeks old, babies begin to relate to, and interact with, their environment. They show increasing interest in exploring the rattle they are given and begin a process of exploration with it, touching it, dropping it, licking it, chewing it and shaking it. This is the early developmental process of making sense of the world around. Babies also begin a process enabling them to interpret facial expression. They begin to respond specifically to their mother's face and to sense or 'read' her feelings, whether they be sad or happy. This will make the baby react in a similar way to the mother's expression. Language and gestures are their bases for feeling secure and safe. If the mother looks very unhappy babies will often respond by crying. If mother looks happy and is chatting to the baby, then the baby will respond by kicking its legs, waving its arms, smiling and gurgling back. This is the beginning of the development of the basic skills of social interaction, and all long before verbal communication develops which further enhances this important interaction between humans that we all value and probably take for granted.

We can probably all recall incidences in an early years setting where a young child is about to embark on a little mischief-making. They may well glance at us first to see if we are looking, and to assess whether to proceed or not. Often a rather stern look will be sufficient to deter them. Through reading our facial expression they know we will be displeased if they proceed and they will be aware of possible consequences they may incur. In a similar situation the child with autism would simply not look at us in the first place. As they are unable to interpret facial expression or even the tone and intonation of verbal interactions, they would see no purpose in looking at us. They may also not be aware of the fact that the intended activity would be deemed as inappropriate or unacceptable in any way.

An additional problem for some children with autism is the inability to interpret emotions or feelings, so the sound of another child crying may cause them a feeling of pleasure and they may become excited and laugh loudly. The fact that the crying child is distressed is not within their comprehension. Unfortunately, this in turn can lead to inappropriate behaviour as they may discover that by pinching a child the result will be that they cry, thus giving them a pleasurable reward. As with any skill or behaviour a young child develops, if they are positively rewarded they are likely to repeat the behaviour unless an alternative behaviour can be established.

In young babies and children, the inability to communicate with the mother is contradictory to all expected bonding processes and can create distance between them if an alternative method of establishing a close relationship is not found. The young child with autism will not be unduly concerned by this lack of bonding as he/she will not have a need to establish such a relationship, but for the mother (and the father) it can be particularly stressful. This could result in their questioning their abilities as a parent, or worse, considering they are a failure as parents. Those parents amongst us will be able to recall the feelings experienced when we went to collect our youngsters from a childminder or nursery – the pleasure on their face, the running towards us with their arms outstretched. This may not be possible for the parent of a child with autism.

The lack of desire to communicate or interact with any other being will also affect the young child in playing with others, either adults or children. By the age of 3 or 4, parallel play (playing alongside another child) is commonplace, and co-operative play (playing interactively with another child) will usually develop. The child with autism will be likely to have developed their own rigid patterns of play that eliminate participation with others, such as lining up cars in exactly the same order over and over again. This child will see no pleasure to be gained from involving another child (or adult) and this question would never arise for them. The desire to play with others simply does not exist. However, playing skills can be developed. This kind of situation can create problems with siblings which would need addressing within the home, but can also be supported by the early years setting.

The lack of desire to play with a wide range of toys and games will also clearly have implications for developing new and progressive skills. For young children, exploring and playing with toys and games presents them with challenges and problems that they need to work out; the accomplishment gives satisfaction, enhances confidence and self-esteem, and motivates the child to continue developing his/her skills. Skills across all developmental areas can progress through constantly exploring the environment and can be further supported by appropriate and timely intervention by an adult to move the child gradually on to the next level. So if a child with autism demonstrates rigid play patterns and does not want to interact with others, then his/her opportunities for developmental progression are clearly compromised. The gap between a young child and his/her peers will widen over the years unless appropriate and meaningful intervention in provided.

Family traditions such as birthdays, religious festivals and celebrations can also be problematic for children and their families as the child with autism may be totally disinterested in the attention received (or not), the celebratory meal, the unusual number of people in the house, the noise level and/or the presents. Celebrating in a church or mosque could also be difficult for the child with autism. The whole event may go unnoticed by the child, or conversely have a severely negative effect resulting in them being very distressed and anxious, evident by screaming, head-banging, rocking, swaying, hand-flapping or similar defensive-type behaviours. To a degree these situations can generally be resolved in resourceful and considerate families but major problems can arise. However, if the situation is resolved by celebrating a low-key and quiet day, then any other children in the family may feel resentful at missing out on the expected frenzy and excitement of the occasion.

Due to the lack of need for interaction with others, the child with autism may resist physical contact with others. The usual cuddling and sharing of a storybook may be of no interest to them unless the book is a part of the child's rigid behaviours. With either adults or other children in the setting, or within the home situation, this could again cause difficulties as others may wish to show the child a book or something in the book which is subsequently ignored. Most children will soon realize this and will simply cease trying, but this is a shame as sharing such an experience should be a pleasurable experience for both parties. Resourceful practitioners and parents can generally overcome such difficulties.

Young children generally enjoy being cuddled, participating in rough and tumble games or football, but if a child with autism feels extreme tactile sensitivity then such experiences can be painful or even excruciating. Even a simple hug could be out of the question and should thus be avoided. Sadly, adults with autism have reported that they were aware they loved some people in their lives but could not understand why this was and admitted even to avoiding handshakes as they were simply too painful. Clearly, once children with autism are able to communicate, either verbally or non-verbally, they can inform us of such issues. Sensory issues will be further explored later in this chapter.

Social interaction is normally further developed through eye contact, so this may help to explain why children with autism avoid eye contact or glance out of the side or corner of their eye. First, they do not wish to interact and, secondly, the experience may be confusing as they may not understand any verbal interaction that follows. Therefore it may be easier to simply avoid the situation.

Although children with autism may not be able to understand someone else's emotions and feelings they do have feelings, and emotions of their own. Despite living in 'a world of their own', that world contains senses, feelings and emotions that we should be aware of. As they become older, children realise they are different and can become very sensitive to the reactions of others. Through a desire to want to participate a child may join in a 'follow the leader' type game but then become confused when the leader changes the actions. If other children laugh or comment, it is then easier to withdraw from the situation and resist trying on another occasion.

CASE STUDY 4.1

Jason is 3 years old and has recently been diagnosed with moderate to severe autism. He has a one-to-one support worker in the early years setting. The social interaction difficulties he experiences include:

- Jason has no desire to play with other children.

- He has no desire to interact with his support worker but walks away when she approaches him.

- Jason stands by the window running his favourite Thomas the Tank Engine back and forth across the window ledge only looking out of the window if an emergency vehicle with the siren blaring goes past.

- If another child takes his toy from him, Jason screams and places his hands over his ears. He can only be calmed by the return of the toy.

- Jason resists invitations to look at or play with alternative activities.

- Jason will not join the rest of the group for snack time and refuses the drink and snack left near him.

- Jason turns away when anyone stands near him and if anyone touches him he screams and flaps his hands.

- Jason has no verbal method of communication.

Case Study 4.1 highlights the nature of the social interaction difficulties of a young child with autism in an early years setting. Jason has clearly been diagnosed with moderate to severe autism and is still at a stage where it is very difficult for practitioners to work with him, due to his lack of interest in any form of interaction, to begin developing his skills and moving him forwards progressively. At this point possible strategies will not be explored, but they will be developed in Chapter 6 when highlighting ways of providing for children with autism. What should be remembered at this stage is that resourceful and well-trained staff will be able to respond to Jason's needs and will be able to provide appropriately to support his future development. Whether all early years settings could accommodate his needs could be an issue for debate. In some areas of the country Jason would attend a special early years unit or school, but in some counties, and with increasing inclusion, more early years settings may be expected to respond to the needs of a child with similar difficulties to Jason.

Social communication

Similarly, reflecting back to Chapter 1, we already have a list of behaviours typically indicative of those experienced by children with autism in the area of social communication.

Children with autism may not develop useful speech at all but remain mute. Some will be able to master a signing system to be used in place of speech, whilst others may not. Some, however, will develop limited speech and language skills, whilst others will develop virtually complete speech and language. Any acquired speech will generally be delayed. So, again, we see that the degree of difficulty in this area will vary from child to child. In addition, and perhaps somewhat more frustrating for parents and families, is the fact that some children may appear to be developing language appropriately and then words may slowly disappear from their vocabulary at the time of regression into the more complex world of autism. For the child with a vocabulary of say, 20 or 30 words, to be able to communicate verbally with those around them and then for the verbalizations to disappear can create a very difficult time for families. To hear your child calling you mummy or daddy is a wonderful feeling, but to be given that pleasure only for it to be removed at a later stage can affect families significantly. Our roles as parents and/or professionals will be to identify, hopefully with the support of a speech and language therapist, ways of moving the child forward from their current, individual stage of development.

The issue of access to speech and language therapy is currently, and has been for many years, an issue of concern to many early years settings. Generally provided by the health department, speech and language therapy will vary according to the type of setting requesting such support, the geographical location and the availability of services in the local authority. Special schools, nurseries, units and classes may be fortunate enough to have their own, or at least a shared, speech and language therapist who attends part time to work with the children and discusses with staff any planned interventions to be used in their absence. Day nurseries, pre-schools groups, nursery schools and classes are more likely to have difficulty in securing the input of a speech and language therapist for a variety of reasons including:

- ■ issues related to funding and budgets – should education or health pay for the service, or if the setting is private should they buy-in such services?

- ■ availability of speech and language therapists – traditionally there have been insufficient available speech and language therapists to fill posts.

It would be hoped that the revised, multidisciplinary Early Years Development and Childcare Partnerships within each county would be able to address such issues and bring an end to a situation that I am aware of that has been ongoing for at least 15 years.

Due to the lack of desire to interact, the young child with autism may not perceive a need to communicate in a verbal manner. Therefore, there would be no reason to learn spoken language. Children with autism may point to something they want, such as a drink or a toy, but will rarely point to show an adult or another child something of interest. The two areas of social interaction and social communication are therefore inextricably linked.

In cases where some speech does develop it may be repetitive, echolalic, unusual and have a monotonous or unusual tone and/or intonation. I have experienced situations where young children with autism have developed echolalic speech (repeating a section of a sentence back to the speaker) but the parents have been so delighted that some speech has appeared that they find it difficult to accept when they are told the speech uttered is meaningless. If a mother asks her child 'Do you want a biscuit?' and the child replies 'Want a biscuit', the parent might interpret this as the child confirming a definite response to the question. In reality the child is simply repeating back the last part of the sentence. There is no evidence to indicate the child has any understanding of the sentence or had, in fact responded to it. It is more likely that the child with autism has heard others responding to questions and assumes some response is necessary. Not understanding the question or how to respond appropriately he/she simply regurgitates some of the sentence and feels that a satisfactory response has been made. The child may feel they are communicating but it is not an effective, meaningful use of speech and language skills.

Children with autism that have difficulties interpreting and making sense of language spoken to them may easily be confused if a person directs conversation towards them. To avoid further confusion some children may react by resorting to stimulatory behaviour such as hand-flapping or covering their eyes or ears, or simply removing themselves from the situation to avoid potential difficulty. As the child becomes older this can clearly create difficulties, as such actions could be interpreted as the child being rude or ignorant, whilst in reality it is a situation-avoidance technique.

The covering of the eyes or ears has always intrigued me, particularly the eyes. The only conclusion I came to whilst working with young children with autism was that this was their attempt to avoid becoming involved with the conversation. By covering the eyes they could try to ignore the fact I was directing speech towards them and, similarly, if they covered their ears this was to stop hearing the communication, thus removing the need for involvement. These suggestions, however, are my own views and are not substantiated by research or other findings.

Some children with autism will develop at least some speech, but the speech may be produced in either an unusual or very monotonous tone, making it difficult to understand or sound interesting. However, this lack of interest is not something that bears significance to the child, only the listener. The speech may also appear disjointed or lacking in flow, with pauses at various points in a sentence. For those working in early years settings and parents alike, this may make it difficult to understand what the child is saying. The additional lack of intonation, from which we derive extra meaning, may further confuse us. To the child with autism, the important point is to utter the words needed. The tone, intonation and interest qualities are irrelevant.

The fact that those with autism invariably fail to interpret facial expression and gestures results in them tending not to use them themselves. If they have no purpose when listening to other people then where is the need to use them yourself when speaking? Again, this can make listening to an autistic child or adult more difficult and parents and practitioners will need to learn to concentrate fully in order to respond appropriately. If the child does not receive appropriate responses to his/her attempts at speech, the result could be that they cease trying.

Due to the repetitive and stereotypical behaviours demonstrated by many children with autism, any speech that develops may be centred on these behaviours, resulting in long, inappropriate and one-sided conversations when the child regurgitates all he/she knows about his/her favourite topic. This can be tedious and at times embarrassing, as the family could be at a social event where such topics are not a part of the conversations taking place. However, the child or adult with autism may simply want to be a part of this conversation that is taking place around him/her and thus interrupt and launch off on their history of perhaps, Thomas the Tank Engine. To interrupt or try to stop them may cause them considerable stress and anxiety, resulting in unacceptable behaviours, so potential difficulties here are evident. Continuing on the inappropriate nature of some verbalizations, some children with autism may learn certain phrases to use at home or in the early years setting but not have an understanding of the meaning attached to them. This could result in them responding to a question such as 'would you like a drink now?' with 'can I leave the table please?' Again, they may be aware that conversation is a two-way process and understand that a question requires a response. Failing to understand the question asked, it is easier to just repeat a known sentence and hope that is sufficient to satisfy the questioner. It is also indicative of a lack of ability appropriately to transfer language learnt in one situation to another situation.

Other children with autism may be unable to understand the conversational process and not really be able to participate appropriately. A child may interrupt someone else who is in the middle of a discussion on books recently read, with, 'the weather's been fine, hasn't it?' Again, this indicates an awareness of the fact that you need to participate in conversations, which can be a pleasant experience, but being unaware of the protocol of conversation that requires we wait until a suitable point before we commence speaking and follow the topic of conversation.

Another difficulty experienced by many children with autism is that of understanding speech in a literal sense only. If we pause to think how many familiar sayings and idioms we use every day, and are now accepted language, we can begin to appreciate how difficult this must be for them. This is further compounded by local dialects and variations, which give us different sayings and phrases in different parts of the country. A useful example of this happened personally some few years ago. My partner asked, when I was washing up, 'Do you want a lift with that?' I replied 'A lift with what? Where am I going?' Confusion ensued until I was able to clarify exactly what he was saying to me. I had not heard this phrase before which in my terminology would be 'Do you want a hand with that?' This same principle would apply to children with autism. Examples of phrases regularly used as a part of everyday life which could confuse a child with autism considerably, would include:

- 'Get your skates on.'   meaning: 'hurry up';

- 'Pull your socks up!'   meaning: 'try harder';

- 'Jump in the bath'   meaning 'Get in the bath' (not jump up and down in the bath);

- 'You're a little angel'   meaning: 'You're a good boy/girl';

- 'Let's have a butcher's'   meaning: 'Let me have a look'.

Parents and practitioners should therefore be careful of the terminology they use in daily life, to avoid possible confusing situations. In a similar vein, children with autism can have great difficulty understanding and interpreting the meaning and purpose of jokes or innuendos in conversation.

Many young children with autism can be encouraged to successfully use alternative methods of communication such as Makaton or Picture Exchange Communication System (PECS). This relieves the pressure created by the inability to converse verbally, as it replaces the verbal element with the use of a sign or pictorial symbol. Many parents have reported that by using such a system the ability to communicate with their child, and for their child to initiate communication with them, has been restored, giving all parties involved great pleasure and satisfaction. Children with autism using Makaton or PECS successfully within both the home and the early years setting can become far less involved in their own 'world' and more an active participant in the world around them. Makaton and PECS will be discussed in more detail in Chapter 5.

Perhaps one of the most useful experiences I have encountered when researching autism has been listening to the words of adults with autism reflecting on their own childhood. Such, now famous, authors as Temple Grandin and Donna Williams are classic examples and I have always felt that I had learnt considerably more from hearing them speak or reading their works than I could from spending a week researching. With specific relation to social communication, hearing Temple Grandin speak increased my understanding of the difficulties experienced by both children and adults. As a world renowned cattle-ranch designer who has gained a PhD, Temple speaks in a slightly monotonous tone and comments that even now in middle age she finds social conversation difficult. She is unable to work out when it is, or is not, appropriate to enter a conversation and often waits so long that the topic of conversation has moved on, causing her some frustration. In a busy social gathering she also has extreme difficulty tuning into one conversation when many other conversations are going on around her. She has to consciously block out some noises and sounds in order to be able to concentrate on one conversation. For this reason she avoids using public telephones in airport lounges as there is a cacophony of background noise and sounds such as planes taking off and landing, public announcements and groups of people holding any number of conversations. It can be so difficult that she cannot hear what the person is saying. This is also related to her heightened sense of hearing, which will be explored later in this chapter. Specifically relating to her early speech development, Temple Grandin recalls:

> *Not being able to speak was utter frustration. If adults spoke to me directly I could understand everything they said, but I could not get my words out. It was like a big stutter … If the therapist pushed too hard I threw a tantrum, and if she did not intrude far enough no progress was made. My mother and teachers wondered why I screamed. Screaming was the only way I could communicate. Often I would logically think to myself, 'I am going to scream now because I want to tell somebody I don't want to do something'. (Internet 8)*

This short extract is significant in helping parents and practitioners to appreciate how it feels to be operating in a world without the ability to speak but with the ability to understand everyone else's speech. Clearly there are implications for practice for parents and practitioners alike.

CASE STUDY 4.2

Emma attends a pre-school setting four sessions a week. She is 3 years old and has been referred to the group by the health visitor who suggests Emma has 'autistic-type behaviours and tendencies'. Emma has been referred to the local child assessment unit for a full developmental assessment. Emma demonstrates the following difficulties in social communication skills:

- Emma avoids direct conversation situations.

- Emma will walk away from an adult or child if they speak directly to her. If they persist, or follow her she will begin to make loud noises, as if trying to drown out the sound, and bang her bricks together. (She always carries six wooden building bricks in her bag which she wears over her shoulder.)

- If encouraged to give eye contact, she will stare at the fluorescent light bulbs suspended from the ceiling.

- If Emma wants a particular toy or snack she will look at it intently, glance at the adult, glance back at the item and so on. This is to indicate her desire for the item.

- Emma can fetch things if an adult points to them, by taking her gaze along your finger and extending her vision to the desired object. If several objects are in the same place she will bring back any object or all of them.

- Emma will respond to her name but only if she feels secure and is confident that she will be able to deal with your request.

As with Case study 4.1 offered earlier in this chapter, strategies to support Emma will be explored in Chapter 6. At this stage it is more important to give the preceding discussion some reality by placing the situation in an early years setting. Again, it should be noted that experienced and resourceful practitioners and parents would be able to respond appropriately to Emma's difficulties.

Imagination

The bulleted list in Chapter 1 gave us a starting point for discussions around difficulties of imagination experienced by children with autism. Seach (1998) succinctly summarizes the complexity of this area:

An impairment in thought and imagination extends to every area of their thinking, language and behaviour. The repetitive and obsessive behaviours can dominate their daily activities and have profound effects on their family and those who work with them. Changes in routine can cause the child distress because they are dependent on routines as a way of understanding the world … It is probably this aspect of the disorder which most profoundly affects how children with ASD are managed both at home and at school. (p. 6)

Play patterns for children with autism tend to be rigid, stereotypical and repetitive, and suggestions for extending this form of play may be strongly resisted. Emma, who was offered in Case study 4.2, would only build with her own bricks. She would take them out of her bag, line them up in a set order, then begin to place one on top of the other. As her fine motor skills improved and became more refined, she would insist that each was squarely seated before attempting to add the next. If when the tower was completed she noticed one was slightly askew, she would place them all quietly back in her bag and repeat the whole process again. Suggestions that she could simply take the tower apart and rebuild it without replacing them in her bag were ignored. If she was encouraged to add one more brick to her collection she would decline, simply, but firmly, saying 'No'. At one point the practitioner attempted to add another brick to her bag without her noticing. This had serious repercussions. She not only spotted the extra brick immediately that she picked her bag up (she always took it off and placed it beside her when she had her drink and snack), presumably from the added weight, but she tipped her bag out onto the nearest table, picked up the offending brick and hurled it across the room, screaming 'No' at the top of her voice. It was clearly very difficult to move Emma away from this rigid behaviour and set pattern of building bricks. If someone demonstrated to her the building of a similar tower but with the bricks in a different order or with an extra brick, she would watch but then become agitated and knock it down. The only other activities Emma engaged in were puzzles – the same puzzles approached in the same way every time – and, interestingly, the sand tray, wherein she would fill up either of the two small buckets with sand and empty them out on her hand, repeating this process over and over. However, she was happy to spend a three-hour session rotating these activities in a routinely rigid manner.

The routine manner of Emma's activities and play are typical of the need for structure and repetition that children with autism need in a world that otherwise is totally confusing. By placing a routine order to events there is security from the chaos. Routines in early years settings are particularly supportive of this difficulty because children will learn the routine and become able to rely on the safety of the known programme of events. Difficulties arise further when routines are broken or disturbed in any way and children with autism should be prepared for changes that are known to be coming in the future. Visits by an outsider can upset routine, as can trips out and even walks to the nearby park. If the room layout is changed to accommodate a new activity, this could also create anxiety and confusion as it upsets the 'normality' these children rely on so heavily. If the running order of the session is altered, perhaps due to the arrival of the annual photographer, then repercussions may occur. The list goes on and on. Perhaps one of the easiest to accommodate is the child's need to drink from the same cup that is used at home, in which case parents could be asked to purchase a spare to be left at the setting for Emma's use.

The resistance to change and need for repetition and familiarity can also extend to food and drink. Children with autism will invariably refuse to try new foods and may have eliminated many items from their diet, sometimes resulting in a very restrictive diet that lacks goodness, vitamins and nourishment, to say nothing of taste. The possible oversensitivity to taste may also affect this area for children with autism as they may be physically sick if a particular food combination or texture is placed in their mouth. Some children with autism will check sandwiches and other foods before placing them in their mouths to ensure the contents are familiar and acceptable. Some children will reject any food combinations such as sandwiches but may eat the components separately.

Such problems can become overdemanding for the family and create many difficulties, such as when shopping for a new bed, the child may have to touch every piece of furniture in the shop and may be resistant to entering in the first place, as it is unfamiliar. If the child will only go into one local supermarket, he/she may only allow the parents to proceed in exactly the same order, going round and insisting that certain items are purchased whether they are needed or not. The impact of such problems is considerable. The above mentioned need to touch all the furniture when moving around a room is evidence of ritualistic behaviour which often accompanies the need for routine and sameness in the life of a child with autism.

A young child with autism may have the ability to see in a picture or object, an unusual aspect that many of us would not otherwise register. This is often linked to other unusual behaviours such as the special liking for one set of toys. A young boy I worked with had a fascination for anything with wheels. Any trains, cars, lorries and other vehicles that he could spot, he would need to explore and possibly involve in his rigid play patterns. His mother had to ensure he was always on reins in his pushchair as he had been known to suddenly fall to the ground to explore the wheels of a passing pushchair or child's tricycle. There are clear indications for concerns by the mother as she stated: 'What on earth will I do when he's too big for the pushchair?' At the same time he could identify the quality of 'roundness' in a whole range of objects in a room or within a picture. They were the only aspects he would generally focus on. He once picked up a soft teddy bear and having turned it around and upside down a few times he stared intently at the facial features. Whilst observing this for the first time I considered many interesting possibilities:

- ■ Was he beginning to extend his restricted play objects to include soft toys or teddy bears? If so, there were implications to introduce other items to him over time.

- ■ Was he learning that inanimate objects were safe to give eye contact to as they would not demand anything of him?

- ■ Was the texture of the fur appealing to him? Again, additional opportunities were coming to mind for future activities with him.

In reality, however, after he repeated the activity several times over the next few days, I became convinced that he had identified the roundness of the bear's eyes and had become fixated with them.

Also allied to social interaction difficulties, children with autism may have difficulties appreciating the perspectives of other people, but this area of difficulty is also linked to lack of imaginative skills. More able children with autism, at the Asperger's syndrome end of the spectrum, may have a more reasonable grasp of someone else's point of view. Within their own lives children with autism consider other people as largely irrelevant so there is no need to be aware of or understand their perspectives and views or to try to understand what they are doing and why. This is also connected to the need for sameness, security and routine as they can only deal with aspects of life that make some sense to them. Familiarity could be threatened by the uncertainty of someone's actions, so for the child with autism it is easier to be unconcerned about other people's actions and intentions.

CASE STUDY 4.3

James was admitted to the nursery class attached to the local primary school. Having been recently diagnosed with autism (moderate) the nursery nurse assigned to work with him has observed the following behaviours that she is particularly concerned about, as she is unsure how to provide for his needs, enabling her to move him forwards developmentally:

■ James will only play with cars and has a set routine to his play. Any attempts to play with him have resulted in displays of anxiety and stress from James, who generally gets up and moves away.

■ James never walks around the room but runs on tiptoe with his hands flapping in front of him, resembling an excited toddler.

■ Doors of any kind fascinate James. On vehicles, in pictures and around the room. He shows more fixated interest if he can open and close them which he will do repeatedly and noisily, laughing at the same time.

■ He will play with the doll's house but only if he first throws all the people and furniture (unless it has doors) onto the floor. He then repetitively opens and shuts the doors, laughing loudly.

■ He shows no interest in any other activities within the playroom. The only time he will touch anything else is when he is exploring it to see if it has a door. Doors govern all his actions and activities.

Case study 4.3 is offered solely to place the preceding discussions in a real situation that any practitioner could be facing, and suggestions for working with James will be explored in Chapter 6. Similarly, although initially it may appear to be an almost impossible situation to have to cope with, experienced and knowledgeable practitioners and parents will be able to respond appropriately to James's needs.

Other behaviours associated with autism

Children with autism may also display one or more of the following behaviours:

■ unusual body movements such as walking on tiptoes, flapping hands (as if excited), rocking and swaying;

■ head-banging, self-biting or other self-injurious behaviour– to the point of causing significant injury;

■ unusual special interests such as knitting or mathematical calculations.

Children with autism who grow up with a special interest may develop exceptional skills in this area despite having severe difficulties in other areas of their development. These skills develop to such a high level of perfection that they would be beyond the capabilities of most people. Such individuals are referred to as *autistic savants*, but they are in the minority. An example is Stephen Wiltshire who has severe learning difficulties in all other areas but can reproduce pencil and watercolour images of buildings with extraordinary brilliance. To see his work is to observe superb artistic quality and when it is considered that he may only see a building for a few minutes and then recall it from memory at a later juncture, the extraordinary nature of this talent becomes evident. Other common savant abilities lie in music and mathematical calculations.

Sensory difficulties

Many children with autism react to sensory stimulation in one of two ways. Either they are oversensitive or undersensitive. This can affect any or all of the sensory areas of touch, vision, hearing, taste and smell. In many cases they develop the ability to block out sounds they do not wish to hear, perhaps for reasons connected with the pitch of the sound being too painful. Whilst research is still taking place in this area, the evidence to date is now building into a considerable and viable explanation for many autistic behaviours, and is also being linked to abnormal development in the brain. Gillingham (1995) explores this area in depth and offers the following insights into the impact of this area of development:

> According to individuals with autism, their disability is linked directly to the senses. They describe how the touch of another human being can be excruciating, smells can be overpowering, hearing can hurt, sight that is distorted, and tastes that may be too strong. The world of the person with autism can be a world of pain. The development of the autistic personality is their method of coping with the pain. (p. 12)

Gillingham continues to offer 'A Sensory Theory of Autism' in which she claims that people with autism find ways to deal with the pain they experience and that the behaviours we see as unusual or odd are in fact their way of coping with the 'pain' of the world around them. She claims that those with autism can produce extra endorphins (biochemicals produced in the brain) by repeating certain behaviours, such as hand-flapping, rocking, covering eyes or ears and so on. The resulting extra endorphins enable the person to create a protective barrier from the pain and effectively block it out. In addition, those with autism develop the ability to overload their senses totally and as a result are able to 'shut down' the sensory system (Gillingham, 1995). This can be achieved through activities such as staring at fluorescent lights and spinning round and round without appearing to become giddy, and head-banging.

Temple Grandin's writing of her experiences as a child with autism substantiates this theory as she explains how she screamed when she could not speak, would hate Sundays as she had to wear her best clothes for church and found them scratchy, 'like sandpaper', and even now, as an adult, has to block out some of her senses selectively in order to cope (Internet 8).

If we reflect back to some of the examples of behaviours demonstrated by young children with autism in this chapter, we can see that sensory explanations do make a good deal of sense. However, we should remain cautious until further and more conclusive research evidence is available.

What can be agreed is that children with autism may demonstrate extremes of sensitivity to the following:

- over/undersensitive hearing – can hear a fire-engine siren before anyone else can;

- oversensitive to or distracted by visual stimuli – such as patterns on curtains or fluorescent lighting;

- over/undersensitive to touch – paper may feel like sandpaper;

- oversensitive to foods and food textures – may not be able to cope with strong or extreme flavours or may be resistant to a variety of flavours tastes and textures.

Considering auditory and visual stimuli is important for early years practitioners as settings are generally well lit, brightly coloured, decorated with colourful displays and busy with sound, all of which can create significant difficulties for children with autism. Clearly, the sensory theory has further implications both for parents and practitioners, which will be further explored in Chapter 6 when we begin to develop ways in which we can support children with autism in the home and the early years setting.

Summary

Throughout this chapter the key areas of difficulty have been examined individually to identify the difficulties experienced by the young child with autism. Combined with the additional reference to the newer sensory theory of autism the real world of the child with autism, has been explored and discussed. The implications for parents and practitioners are considerable, as without this knowledge I would reiterate my concern that individuals may be compounding a child's difficulties when they in fact consider they are helping the child to move forwards and develop new skills. If parents and practitioners are not fully aware of the many ways in which children with autism can behave, then they cannot ensure their provision is appropriate and meeting the child's needs. For example, we can understand that the sudden flapping of hands and jumping up and down is not simply an unusual behaviour but the way a child copes with a situation that he/she feels is threatening, confusing or creating pain. With this heightened awareness and knowledge of the world of the autistic child it is hoped that parents and practitioners will be better placed to cope with and provide effectively for individual needs. Ways in which we can adapt our provision and strategies to support children with autism will be explored in a subsequent chapter.

Key issues

■ *Parents and practitioners need to have considerable knowledge of the effects of autism on the children they support in order to provide effectively.*

■ *This raises issues of training, access to training and therefore funding, as all early years practitioners should have access to such training and information.*

■ *The issues of access to and equity of access to speech and language therapy services should be resolved.*

■ *With appropriate knowledge early years practitioners can respond to the individual needs of young children with autism.*

Some suggestions for discussion

Item 1
In the light of information gathered from this chapter, reflect on Case study 4.1 of Jason. As a staff consider ways in which you could provide for Jason's needs.

Item 2
Consider a child you are currently working with or have worked with in the past and list the key behaviours they demonstrated in the areas of: social interaction, social communication, imagination. Identify any changes you may have made to your provision in the light of new knowledge gained from reading this chapter.

Item 3
Reflect on the training needs of staff within your setting with regard to providing for children with autism. If it is considered that additional training is needed, try to identify ways to proceed.

📖 Suggested further reading

Gillingham, G. (1995) *Autism. Handle with Care!* Texas: Future Horizons.

Siegel, B. (1996) *The World of the Autistic Child: Understanding and Treating Autistic Spectrum Disorders.* Oxford: Oxford University Press, Chapters 2, 3 and 4.

Website – Temple Grandin: www.autism.org/temple/inside.

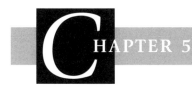

CHAPTER 5

Programmes of intervention

Introduction

Having explored definitions of autistic spectrum disorders and discussed the areas of difficulty that the young child with autism may be experiencing, we need to begin to develop ways in which these young children can best be supported. In this chapter some of the more well-known programmes of intervention will be debated.

To provide effectively for a child's needs the initial diagnosis combined with an understanding of the family perspective and the very individual needs of their child with autism need to be thoroughly assessed. At this point it should become clearer as to which approach, or approaches, and strategies will be most useful for that particular child. At all times practitioners and parents should remember that every child with autism will have different needs, so one blanket programme for all children with autism will not be appropriate.

Knowledge of existing programmes should give practitioners and parents a broad overview of those that may be available to them and, when they consider the child in question, it should become apparent that some approaches would be more suitable for the child than others. All approaches will have merits but matching each one to the individual child should inform subsequent decisions.

Practitioners and parents should also consider that there are no guarantees with programmes of intervention and there are occasions when it is more appropriate for an individual child to work on a tailor-made programme following discussions between parents and professionals. Nobody should feel compelled to take on board an intervention package unless they are as certain as they can be that it will have positive outcomes for the child.

Early intervention

There is ample evidence to support the notion of early identification for all children experiencing difficulties. For children with autism it is equally as important, if not more so. Parents of children with autism have reported that despite having already fought long and hard to secure a diagnosis, the gap between that, time and appropriate intervention or support is, 'for most parents and families, a distressing experience' (NAS,1999a, p. 1). Having received the diagnosis, parents and families need clear and sound advice and guidance to proceed as soon as possible to establishing effective intervention and the beginnings of future progress. The Department for Education and Skills (DfES) document, *Intervening Early*, supports the need for early intervention: 'By intervening at an early stage, the downwards spiral, where difficulties get worse, become harder to address, and lead to failure, can be prevented' (2002, p. 3). From the parental perspective, Bill Davis (2001) states that: 'Early intervention is the single most important concept in treating autism' (p. 59). He continues to highlight the need for immediate action and advises parents not to wait until the time of school entry.

Trevarthen et al. (1998) further pinpoint the value of early intervention:

> *Preschool children with autism can, with responsive, specialist help to aid them with communication difficulties, be attracted to form relationships and learn cooperative behaviours by involving them in educational games similar to those used with their unaffected peers, and the company of other young children, with their direct approaches and enthusiasm, can help in this. (p. 169)*

It therefore becomes clear that parents and professionals need access to relevant information to advise and guide them in the range of approaches available for their child. This will enable them to begin constructive and appropriate strategies with the child. It is fundamental at an early stage to plan and implement strategies that will encourage the development of interaction, communication and imagination skills (the triad of impairments), and as play is such a powerful medium for learning, it would appear logical that any such strategies should be play based. Activities using the child's preferred interests and where possible the child's preferred resources are most likely to be successful. For example, if a child displays rigid and repetitive play routines with trains, then trains would be an appropriate focus for the practitioner- or parent-devised activities. Results will not be immediate but with patience and flexibility, a well-planned, structured and gradual system will, in my own experience, reap rewards in time. Once the young child is able to tolerate the adult's closer presence real progress can begin.

Specific approaches

The range of programmes to support children with autism and their families seems to grow almost by the month. The programmes outlined below are perhaps the most well known, with a few lesser-known programmes also included. Due to limitations of space only a brief overview of each is offered but suggested reading and a list of contact details is included at the end of the chapter for those wishing to find out more.

Lovaas

The Lovaas approach is a form of applied behavioural analysis in which the Lovaas trainer models to the child a skill to be mastered, such as placing one brick on top of another, and then encourages the child to replicate. This technique is undertaken by qualified trainers who generally sit at a child-sized table with the child opposite and facing. Eye contact is requested using a prompt of tilting or directing the child's head if necessary, and the request for the child to complete the task is repeated until success is achieved. Success is always positively rewarded, often by a small item of favoured food and activity-specific verbal feedback, such as 'Good brick building!' For the child who fails or does not wish to attempt the task, a firm verbal comment can be made, such as 'No!'

The Lovaas programme is totally adult led with the adult selecting the activity and materials to be used. The programme is based on the behavioural theory that children are likely to repeat learned behaviours that are positively rewarded and less likely to repeat behaviours that are negatively rewarded.

Reports indicate that young children with autism can be resistant initially to such a rigid and adult-led approach as their world does not include participation with others, adults or children, neither do they wish to play with adult-selected activities, especially activities structured and led by anyone but themselves. In the early stages this may result in bouts of continued screaming and constantly leaving their seat. The trainer would reposition the child at the table..

Until such time as the child can interact socially with others the Lovaas programme will generally be undertaken in the home by a team of trained Lovaas workers who will work regularly with the child. It is hoped that the child's parents will observe and become more involved with the programme as time progresses. The activities are highly structured and would be planned individually for the child, responding directly to individual needs. Reports suggest that many children achieve considerable success within the programme and some are able to proceed to mainstream provision.

Opponents to such a programme for very young children could suggest that it does not take into account the reasons why the children do not wish to participate or to involve themselves in adult-selected activities. In addition, the child's reactions are their way of trying to cope with the anguish and difficulties created within themselves by this structured approach. It could also be suggested that such an approach will teach skills in a 'robotic' fashion and, although the child may be able to complete tasks or a set of learned skills successfully, they may have difficulties transferring the skills to another situation. Similarly the approach does not support the development of imagination, as the adult is doing the thinking, and deciding, for the child. Some professionals have questioned the methodology and therefore the validity of the research originally undertaken by Lovaas in 1987, which claimed to indicate the positive outcomes of the programme. However, due to the difficulties of undertaking research with children with autism, attempts to replicate the study have been unsuccessful.

Parents taking on board such an intensive programme would require patience, stamina and the ability to be available for considerable periods each week to participate. For many parents whose children are working on the programme they would suggest that as the programme can be started early when the child is at the pre-school stage, it is worth the commitment needed and reaps good rewards.

Treatment and Education of Autistic and Related Communication Handicapped Children

The TEACCH programme was developed in North Carolina and was developed to address the need for children and adults with autism to have structure and routine in their lives. The programme begins at the pre-school phase and continues through to adulthood, with the hope that many of the TEACCH students will then be able to hold down purposeful employment within the local community. Developed by Eric Schopler and his team at the university, there are certain key principles underpinning the programme:

- structured environment;
- work schedules;
- work systems;
- visual instructions.

The programme is established in the setting or school and is also followed at home and within the community, therefore ensuring consistency in the child's life. Due to the difficulties experienced with children with autism trying, and generally failing, to make sense of the so-called 'normal' world, the TEACCH programme offers a 'world' that is understandable to the child. Through this methodology the child can function more independently and apply themselves to learning more effectively.

In a typical TEACCH classroom each area would be distinctly separated from other areas with screens or cupboards, this signifies to the child what happens in each area, offering clarity of understanding. Individual children will have their own timetable or 'work schedule' to work from which will initially be in pictorial form. Often running from top to bottom, each schedule will have the child's name, and possibly a symbol belonging to that child for ease of recognition, so that each child knows which is their schedule. On arrival the child would take the first picture and go to the table (and area) where he/she knows that activity takes place, placing their schedule card in a tray or box at the start so that teachers can check to see which areas each child has visited. On the table there will be a box with the child's name placed at the left-hand side of the table, which the child picks up and opens. Whatever is inside is the task for completion in that work area. When the task has been completed the box will be placed on the right-hand side of the table to indicate it is finished. The child goes back to the work schedule, takes the next picture off the work schedule and proceeds to that area of the room, and so on. During each session there is little change to this routine so the child feels secure within the environment and is happy to undertake the tasks set with a degree of independence.

At some point the teachers will work one to one with each child to begin learning new skills, complete new tasks or assess progress. The children readily accept this involvement. The work table will be in a distraction-free area, perhaps facing a wall without bright posters and stimulating images to distract the child, or being able to see the other children moving around the room. This supports the fact that children work and concentrate better in sensory-free areas that will not overstimulate the senses. The moving of the boxes on the table from the left to the right is significant and is always performed in this manner, to aid understanding of left–right orientation, as will be required later in reading and writing. In addition, the tasks contained within the boxes are child specific, in that if the teacher wants the child to match five pictures to one picture strip, then only the five pictures and the one strip will be in the box. The child is then clear regarding exactly what is expected for successful completion of the task without needing support, thus gaining independence.

As a child becomes more able the schedules and instructions for the tasks will be produced pictorially and in words, until such a time as the child is hopefully able to use solely the written word. Within the home environment the family is expected and encouraged to adopt the same principles to enable the child to function more fully as a family member. This would even extend to the family being able to go to a restaurant for a meal, taking with them, or leaving behind at the restaurant, the child's familiar cutlery, crockery, napkins and glassware. This way the child feels more secure and is less likely to react negatively to being in an unusual environment full of new and confusing items. As the TEACCH programme extends to the community as well, this is accepted practice within some shops and restaurants within the towns of North Carolina, and participating establishments would normally be happy to support families in this way. The TEACCH approach is designed to advise and support parents and the community as much as possible through working closely with them.

The structure given to children offers them a more stable life, safe in the knowledge of what is happening next and what will be expected of them. Some young children may scream, rock, sway and/or head-bang if a parent tries to put their coat on them. This could be due to the fact that the child does not understand what will happen next. If however the child is using a timetable or schedule within the home, then he/she will be aware of what happens next and is less likely to react in the same way.

Through this highly structured environment it is claimed that children are more able to apply themselves to the learning situation and thus make greater progress. Whilst the programme may feel overstructured and thus limit individual thought and imagination, these skill areas are also addressed within the curriculum.

The TEACCH approach is now widely used in the USA and some European countries. One area of England has adopted the TEACCH approach and many education staff are now TEACCH trained. Therefore, children with autism can generally be accommodated in mainstream schools and early years settings. TEACCH training courses are available in the UK but are costly, thus possibly prohibiting participation by voluntary sector practitioners. Those working in self-funding establishments would not generally have the financial means to support such expense.

Problems could arise if a family moves into another county or country where the TEACCH approach is not used, which could create considerable anxiety for the child and family. In addition, overreliance on structures may demand structure in every aspect of a person's life, which is clearly not always practical. However, the community-wide aspect of this approach is beneficial, as is the structured approach, which enables the child with autism to participate more fully in a world that otherwise causes them considerable anxiety and stress. Parents and practitioners should remember, however, that one approach is not necessarily a panacea for all children. Whilst the TEACCH approach may be highly relevant to some, or even the majority, of children with autism, it may not be appropriate for all.

Daily Life Therapy (Higashi)

Originating in Japan, but now established in America, Daily Life Therapy provides group activities based on the following aims:

- ■ improved physical strength through regular and strenuous group exercise activities which reduces anxiety and introduces structure and routine;

- ■ stimulation of the child's intellectual interest and development;

- ■ conformity to accepted social behaviours;

- ■ a positive ethos of success and encouragement;

- ■ key principle: to create the 'rhythm of life' in the children.

Pupils can either board, or attend daily, and although it is a costly exercise, parents report that considerable improvements are evident in physical skills, a reduction of inappropriate behaviours and improvements in self-help skills such as eating, washing and toileting. Some children from the UK have been to the school, many of whom were funded by the local authority. However, this option would not be available to all parents who might feel it is the most appropriate provision for their child.

The children are not formally taught a curriculum that would match or link in with the National Curriculum and concerns have been raised about the abilities of the children to transfer skills learnt within the physical structure of the school once they have left. Communication skills are not taught as a separate area but all instructions use verbal communication, with no forms of signing being used. This could be perceived as a major difficulty, as the success of alternative communication approaches have been well documented. In addition, as all the children are taught in groups, one might question the appropriateness of the curriculum which neither responds to individual needs, nor encourages freedom of choice and the development of imaginative skills. However, research does support the use of regular physical exercise for children with autism, as it has been shown to reduce inappropriate behaviours and anxiety.

Son-Rise programme (options approach)

The Son-Rise programme was developed by the Kaufmans in America as the result of their own work with their son from about 18 months. Now an adult, his parents claim he has improved so dramatically that he no longer has autism. Through a belief in accepting and loving the child for who he was, and for what he had to offer, the Kaufmans developed a separate playroom for the programme to work in. After initiating the programme and seeing successes they then recruited friends and volunteers to help them, as they believed that ideally the child should be with a mentor for the whole day and evening, that is, as long as he was awake. The principle of helping the child to learn what he/she wants to learn, as opposed to what others may want him/her to learn or what is perceived to be needed, is fundamental. The mentor will undertake a range of activities combining following the child's own lead and participating in whatever they are doing (as a way of indicating acceptance of their play) and encouraging the child to participate in adult-selected activities. Observation is regularly undertaken, of both the child and the mentor, often through a two-way mirror, and the mentors meet regularly to plan future activities.

In the past, families from the UK have had to fund their own trip to the Son-Rise centre in America to undergo a period of training, usually up to a month. On their return to England they could remain in touch with the centre by email, telephone and sending videos of activity sessions for feed-back by the specialist trainers in America. However, quite recently the Options centre has opened an additional centre in London, which will clearly reduce the financial implications. Parents are, however, expected to set up their own playroom to run the activity sessions in, which is free from dis-tractions and totally child focused.

Questions spring to mind about the exclusive nature of such an approach, which would limit considerably contact with other children and family members. This also has implications relating to adaptation to other set-tings and environments. Is the child then able to go on family outings, to the shops or the park? The sheer intensity of interacting with a rota of adults for the majority of your waking hours is also somewhat unnatural and would not seem to support the development of socially acceptable behaviours or trans-ference of skills learnt.

SPELL (National Autistic Society)

The SPELL approach was devised by the National Autistic Society and is used within their own independent, boarding and day schools throughout the UK. The NAS (2001) states the aim of the approach is: 'To provide a broad and balanced curriculum that takes account of the pupil's autism and learning needs and teaches independence and life-enhancing skills and experiences. Access to the National Curriculum is incorporated into individually-designed programmes' (p. 48). Through the individually tailored programmes each child will be taught in small classes using structure, routine, consistency of approach and low levels of distraction. As this approach is associated with the NAS, the staff will be trained in the nature of autism, effects of autism and the implications for the child and the teacher. Whenever possible, children would attend such a school as a measure to support specialist teaching but with a view to returning to their local mainstream school.

The name SPELL is derived from elements that are representative of the approach:

Structure – which helps reduce anxiety and stress and creates security within the child's classroom environment.
Positive attitudes to success and expectations that are achievable and realistic yet still supporting development.
Empathy – through understanding the world and the difficulties of the child with autism.
Low arousal – an environment free from too many distractions to enable the child to access the curriculum and achieve maximum learning.
Links – with parents, schools, the community and other professionals involved with the child and/or family.

The fundamental principles of this approach are clearly embedded in a thorough understanding and knowledge of issues related to young children with autism, and clearly this is a major strength of the approach. As NAS schools are inspected by OFSTED, there is accountability, plus the knowledge that the children will have been working within the National Curriculum wherever appropriate, thus supporting transfer back to mainstream schools. It is assumed that a period of transition would be incorporated into the transfer to local schools, as mainstream staff would need to have some knowledge of the most appropriate provision to continue supporting the child's individual needs, in an accessible way for the child that is also manageable for the staff. The NAS is undertaking their own research, through following the progress of the children, but other research evidence is not readily available.

Early Bird (National Autistic Society)

Beginning in 1997 the Early Bird approach was established to support pre-school children with autism by training their parents (or a close family member) over a three-month period. This form of early intervention gives parents knowledge and understanding of the impact of autism on their child, and subsequently their family. By attending weekly meetings parents meet other parents, which offers additional support, and learn strategies to use with their child to support their development in the key areas of communication, interaction and imagination. In addition, strategies to cope with difficult behaviours are also discussed. The programme can be used by any professionals working with young children with autism who undertake the Early Bird training. This ensures that the necessary skills are acquired to take back to their local area and begin their own programme of training for parents. Shields (2000) reports:

> They learn how to set up and run the programme, with the help of the extensive supporting materials: the Early Bird Training Manual, video, and Parent book, multidisciplinary teams have already been trained, with skill mixes including that of specialist health visitor, and funding for training applications is coming from a range of sources. (p. 54)

The programme uses aspects of the Hanen programme, which teaches parents approaches to supporting the speech and language and social skills of their children, and TEACCH programmes and has three key strands:

- understanding autism;
- development of strategies to improve the child's communication and interaction;
- analysing behaviours to enable parents to reduce unacceptable behaviours.

As the programme is still in comparative infancy, there is little research evidence available to support the success or otherwise of the programme. However, the fact that the underpinning principles are based on sound knowledge of autism would be indicative of its usefulness, particularly as parents of pre-school children may find it otherwise difficult to obtain autism-specific support and intervention. The availability of such a programme to all parents in the UK who would wish to use it would be an issue of current concern, but presumably as more trainers are available, wider access to the Early Bird programme will follow. Currently, Portage, a home-based developmental intervention programme, may be the only more widely available approach.

Speech and language therapy

Due to the specific training needed, only speech and language therapists should undertake assessments of the speech and language development of a young child with autism. Due to the difficulties being specifically related to social communication this is possibly more likely to succeed if undertaken in small groups or within the early years setting, as opposed to individual treatment sessions. Speech and language therapists should, however, have a thorough understanding of the difficulties experienced by children with autism and their need for an effective system of communication with which they can begin to interact with the world. For this purpose PECS and Makaton are commonly used. The speech and language therapist would work closely with the staff of the setting, assisting with the development of appropriate interventions and activities.

PECS (Picture Exchange Communication System)

This system has, in my own experience, been very successful with young children with special needs, and particularly with children with autism. The system is based on the principle of involving the child in communication by offering them opportunities to request items, which is not a skill young children with autism feel they have a need for. As an example, if at snack time we were offering a child milk or water to drink, all children would generally be expected to choose and ask for their drink. Two pictures, one of a glass of milk, the other of water, would be available to the child with autism. The child would learn to select the card indicating the preferred drink and give it to the adult by way of a request. The adult would then praise the child and repeat the request verbally to model appropriate language, such as: 'You would like a glass of milk. Well done!' The system is not intended to replace speech, rather that it should reduce the frustration of being unable to communicate, offer correct models of speech and language, and give the child increased independence.

Initially, two adults would be needed to teach the basic concept to the child. The cards would be placed in front of the child, with the first adult offering the two drinks to the child. The second adult would show the child the picture of the favoured drink, place it in their hand and help them to give it to the other adult. This indicates the child's need to take responsibility for the decision and the request. Since the evolution of PECS it has become widely used in pre-school settings and schools. As well as enabling interaction and non-verbal speech between the child and the adults, the benefits also extend to the home and to other children within the setting who can also be approached by the child with autism to request something. As the child becomes more competent with a few basic pictures, then more and more words can be introduced, building to sentence structure and phrases, if appropriate.

Although concerns may be raised about the child then having no need to develop verbal speech and language, research so far indicates the opposite to be true. In time, language is likely to develop due to the pressure to learn and use verbal communication having been removed. Consistently hearing correct language models supports the gradual development of language.

Makaton

Makaton is a basic signing system, with each sign having a matching line drawing to give pictorial support. Due to the nature of the difficulties of young children with autism, the signing itself may be problematic for some, but the clear pictures used are highly appropriate because of their preference for visual clues. Used as a method to support and clarify understanding by the child, Makaton can be used both in the early years setting and the home, if parents are supportive. Similar to the PECS system, Makaton is not intended to replace speech, but to enable a child who has no other form of communication to begin developing such skills. Many early years practitioners, especially those working in special schools, nurseries and assessment centres, will be trained to use Makaton. These practitioners tend to use signs and language whenever they are communicating with the children in the setting, even if some of the children have developed, or are developing, language. Other children in the setting then tend to pick up the signs as well, thus enabling further help to the child with autism and the opportunity to begin their own, direct form of communication and interaction. When using Makaton, only key words are generally signed, but where appropriate, signs for each word can be used. Training over several days by a Makaton trainer is available in most parts of the UK.

Sensory integration

Working on the principle that children with autism have difficulties receiving and interpreting sensory information appropriately, sensory integration aims to redress this imbalance through the use of sensory stimulation. Multi-sensory rooms are available in some early years settings in the UK, where children can enjoy the range of stimulating materials available, through their own exploration. These could include visual, tactile and auditory stimuli. Physical exercise, sometimes led by physiotherapists or occupational therapists, such as swimming and movement, can also help to stimulate the child's physical skills. The approach is used to enable children to interpret sensory stimulation in a more appropriate manner by reducing both hyper- and hypo-sensitivity to the stimuli, which in turn supports progress in communication, interaction, imagination and thus enables learning.

However, if we reflect back to Gillingham's sensory development work discussed in Chapter 4, it could be suggested that overstimulation can create anxiety and stress in children with autism. This links with elements of approaches such as TEACCH and SPELL that recommend children work in areas that are free of sensory stimuli, in order to concentrate more fully on the task in hand. It will therefore depend on the practitioner's level of knowledge about autism and the individual children, combined with their ability to use sensory stimuli in a carefully planned way.

Facilitated Communication

Facilitated Communication (FC) is an approach designed to support communication through the use of a facilitator and a computer keyboard, pictureboard or a normal range of pictures attached to a thick board. The facilitator will support the child's arm or wrist above, or in front of, the keyboard, but the child will make the connection with the board to indicate a word, or several words representing a phrase or sentence. This method can be used with children with a range of special needs, including those with autism.

The main question raised over the use of FC is how to ensure the communication is the direct result of the child's input as opposed to the facilitator's inadvertent guiding of the child's arm and pre-empting what the child may wish to communicate. Although it is hoped that the child will develop greater independence using this method, there are some children who are not able to develop any degree of independence, relying on the presence of a familiar facilitator to communicate, which is clearly not always practical.

Auditory Integration Training

Auditory Integraton Training (AIT) is an approach developed independently by Tomatis and Berard, French physicians, who both worked on the principle that children with autism may have distorted hearing. Through the use of auditory stimulation they considered the brain could be adjusted to interpret sounds more appropriately and to block out unwanted sounds.

The specific areas of auditory difficulty are pinpointed through an initial audiogram that will be repeated at the end of the treatment. It is hoped that the final audiogram would indicate normal or near normal auditory function. Depending on the results of the initial audiogram, specific sounds, tones and pitch levels will be fed through headphones to the child on a daily basis for a period of about ten days. Reports by AIT teachers and parents indicate good outcomes, but clearly their direct involvement with the approach would cast questions of bias and thus the validity of their feedback. The cost of such treatment may be prohibitive to some parents, particularly as local authorities are not generally supportive of funding alternative approaches.

Information and communications technology (ICT) education and therapy

Now that computers are in so many early years settings and homes, and we are all living in a computerized world, the educational value of computer-assisted learning is evident. Young children adapt to computers from a very young age and some are far more competent than their parents by the end of the primary stage of education. For children with autism it may be easier to interact with a computer than other people. The computer is non-threatening so does not generally create anxiety (unless it crashes). Once a child is used to a new application, he/she will know clearly what is expected, thus offering no confusion, giving the child control, opportunities to put right any mistakes and without the need for verbal interaction. The computer can therefore be used to support the child's developments across all skill areas, although practitioners should be cautious about overuse by children with autism, as it can be a very solitary activity. Children also need opportunities to develop their interaction and communication skills. Murray (1997) contends that:

> Information technology offers scope to play, explore, be creative, in a safe, highly controllable environment – and it need not make any verbal demands. Computers can thus focus attention with minimal risk of overload. They may also provide various coping strategies for people with problems of self-awareness, information connection and memory retrieval. (p. 100)

Play therapy

The area of play and its importance when providing for young children with autism will be further explored in Chapter 6. However, most early years practitioners would acknowledge and support the value of play-based learning, which is further supported by the government's Early Learning Goals (QCA, 1999) and Foundation Stage Curriculum for the Early Years (QCA, 2000). The implications for, and benefits of, play-based learning for children with autism should be evident once barriers to interaction have been overcome.

If we reflect briefly on the difficulties related to play that children with autism experience, we will be able to see that whilst a play-based approach is useful, knowledge and understanding of these specific difficulties is essential to inform planning and thus enable progress for the child. The difficulties include:

- use of senses when exploring items, e.g. licking, tasting, feeling;

- stereotypical and rigid play patterns;

- focus on unusual parts of items being explored;

- long periods of time spent repeating the same play activity;

- lack of direct eye contact, e.g. using peripheral vision to inspect items;

- lack of attention and concentration on adult-led tasks;

- lack of imaginative, functional or symbolic play;

- tendency to repeat learned play patterns.

Rather than attempting to have a play-based curriculum to enable learning, the child with autism therefore needs to be taught to play. With increased practice it is hoped that an effective play therapy approach would lead to independent and imaginative play by the child. Key skills that can be supported would be imitation, turn-taking, social interaction and cognitive skills. Through play strategies that are individually planned for the child, combined with the observation and assessment of play skills, considerable progress can be made.

Music therapy

This approach aims to enable interaction and communication through music and the use of musical instruments. Without the need for verbal communication it can be a pleasant and rewarding experience for children with autism, as their limited communication skills are not needed. The therapist would be specially trained, in what has become a registered profession, and would plan to accommodate individual needs during the sessions. The session could aim to develop skills in turn-taking, eye contact, self-awareness, feelings and emotions, and the establishing of a relationship between the child and therapist.

One of the great advantages is that whilst the therapist will be working towards developing skills, the child will take the lead in many activities with the adult responding to their actions. It is therefore a non-confrontational and non-threatening situation for the child.

Trevarthen et al. (1998) devote a whole chapter to describing and analysing music therapy and offer the reader detailed documentary evidence by way of a case study of a 3-year-old called 'Colin'. Through analysing video and audio evidence the authors provide an in-depth and accessible introduction to the theory and benefits of music therapy. The authors conclude that: 'musical interaction helps autistic children to gain a self-awareness and relatedness to others – an awareness and relatedness that is cohesive rather than fragmented, enabling them to respond more readily in everyday social interaction' (ibid., p. 202).

Art therapy

Few would contest the therapeutic value of art. It is a way of expressing oneself and of communicating in a safe way where there are no correct or incorrect answers. Whatever you create, and in whatever medium, should be respected and valued by those who view it. Therefore, the benefits of art therapy with young children with autism should not be overlooked.

Having observed young children with autism experimenting with paint, often hesitantly at first as they did not seem to comprehend what the experience was about, I have seen a child hold the paintbrush vertically, and simply watch the paint trickle down the brush handle, onto his hand and down his arm. The sensory experience was clearly being enjoyed. This particular child then proceeded to make his impression with the paint on his hand and arm, transferring it onto the paper, yet discarding the brush. I then sat next to him and imitated his actions, commenting on the way it felt and making my own marks on my paper. This shared experience was successful in both social interaction and communication, as well as being an enjoyable creative and sensory experience.

Drama and dance therapy

Drama and dance therapy can be used in many ways with children with autism. Music can be played either by an adult or via a tape recorder or radio, and the children, plus any adults available, can proceed to move freely around the room. Alternatively, a session could be planned to include more structured elements. Any such experiences will again support the development of social interaction and communication but will also benefit physical skills. The sensory aspect of the experience will also benefit the child with autism. Trained dancers or dance and drama therapists would be welcomed in settings providing for children with special needs, including children with autism.

Dietary and vitamin treatments

Research evidence undertaken regarding the benefits of changes to diet and/or the use of vitamin supplements is overall inconclusive. Within the whole population there are a small percentage of people who experience certain food allergies or intolerances, often citing wheat and dairy products as problematic. It would therefore seem appropriate to consider that a similar percentage of children with autism are likely to experience such difficulties. In addition, some children with autism have a tendency to difficulties with their digestion and bowels, leading to constipation or diarrhoea. With the support of a dietician and under paediatric supervision, elimination of foods can be suggested as a way to assess possible food intolerances, but as children with autism can often have problems with food, due to their taste, texture and smell sensitivities, this could prove difficult.

Paul Shattock, at the Autism Research Unit in Sunderland, has undertaken considerable research in the area of food allergies and intolerances in children with autism, and has suggested that a gluten- and dairy-free diet has resulted in considerable benefits, particularly for those at the more severe end of the spectrum.

Choosing a programme of intervention

With such a range of approaches available, and the list was not exhaustive, it is clear that parents will need support and advice on choosing a programme for their child. What should always be remembered is that parents know their child better than anyone else and, when that knowledge is combined with the expertise of the practitioners who have been working with their child, an informed decision should become a little easier. Parents should be advised against paying too much attention to the 'miracle cures' as seen in the media on a fairly consistent basis, and should rely on their own good sense and knowledge to make this important decision. Of course, it is not compulsory that parents must choose one of the options available, as the local early years setting may offer outstanding provision for young children with autism, based on a thorough underpinning knowledge of the effects and implications of autism for the child, the family and the setting and how best to provide for the difficulties of the child. Children with autism, as stated previously, like all children, are unique and individual. The programme that is more appropriate for one child will not necessarily be the most appropriate for the next child. In addition, parents will need to reflect on more practical issues such as which programmes are available in their locality, what cost (if any) would be incurred, how it would affect the family, levels of involvement and commitment needed, and so on.

Settings demonstrating effective provision for young children with autism may use elements of more than one approach mentioned within this chapter and not restrict themselves to the confines of one singular programme, offering a more eclectic approach. Personally, I used key elements of TEACCH plus some elements of sensory theory, combined with a play-based developmental curriculum similar to that described by writers on play therapy. This approach, when adapted to individual strengths and preferences, and taking into account the difficulties experienced by each individual child, appeared to work well with the children I supported. This is, of course, simply a suggestion, which is unsupported by research evidence.

Although the range of programmes offered within this chapter is considerable, when carefully examined, some key factors emerge that appear to support development and progress in young children with autism in a generic way.

Common features of effective programmes of intervention

Provision for young children with autism can only be effective if the practitioners have knowledge of autism and how to provide effectively. They should therefore have a thorough underpinning knowledge of:

- the effects of autism on the child;

- an understanding of the world of the young child with autism;

- the impact of autism on the child, the family, the practitioner and the setting;

- knowledge of a range of intervention programmes;

- appropriate training for all staff members on the difficulties the children may experience and effective strategies to support them;

- thorough understanding of child development;

- knowledge of and expertise in effective observational techniques;

- expertise in planning to respond to individual needs.

Once the practitioner is skilled and experienced, the key features of effective practice would be evident in their daily work. These are likely to include:

■ early intervention;

■ close and effective partnerships with parents;

■ close and effective partnerships with allied professionals;

■ structure and routine for the child;

■ use of visual clues to support the child;

■ inclusion of one-to-one teaching situations;

■ regular observation;

■ adaptation to accommodate individual needs;

■ awareness of sensory issues;

■ work areas that are lacking visual stimulation;

■ planning which includes consideration of the child's preferences and strengths as well as difficulties;

■ the development and use of autism-specific strategies to promote learning for the child.

Discussion of issues of effective practice will be further developed in chapter 6.

Summary

A wide range of programmes of intervention has been offered for consideration within this chapter, with many of them using similar strategies to develop skills. What becomes evident is that one programme alone will be unlikely to meet all the needs of all children with autism. Each child should be viewed as individual with decisions based on parental and practitioner knowledge. Combined with effective parental and multidisciplinary partnerships, we would then be in a good position to provide appropriately for the young child with autism. This view is supported by Howlin (1998):

> Those programmes that have proved most successful acknowledge the variety and pervasiveness of the deficits in autism and accept the need to employ a range of different techniques. There are no magic answers, no 'quick fixes', no infallible recipes. Instead, the choice of treatment will

depend on individual patterns of skills and abilities, as well as family circumstances, all of which will influence the ways in which various techniques or strategies can be employed. (p. 101)

Key issues

- *A range of diverse approaches is available for consideration but no single programme is likely to address the needs of all young children with autism.*

- *Parents will need advice and guidance from knowledgeable practitioners.*

- *All practitioners need knowledge, expertise and skills in providing for children with autistic spectrum disorders.*

- *Equity of access to training for all practitioners is needed.*

- *Equity of access to programmes for all parents is needed.*

Some suggestions for discussion

Item 1
If you are currently providing for a young child with autism, reflect on the range of intervention programmes offered within this chapter and consider if any may be appropriate, or if elements might be used.

Item 2
Reflect on the ways in which guidance and advice is given to parents. Do you have accessible information for parents on the range of programmes available? If not, could this, and should this, be addressed? Formulate ways of developing this.

Item 3
Consider the issues parents have to address when faced with considering options for their child. Write a list of factors you would recommend they consider.

Item 4
Are all staff members adequately trained in all areas of providing for young children with autism? If not, identify ways to support future developments in this area.

📖 Suggested further reading

Cumine, V., Leach, J. and Stephenson, G. (2000). *Autism in the Early Years: A Practical Guide*. London: David Fulton, Chapter 4.

Jones, G. (2002) *Educational Provision for Children with Autism and Asperger Syndrome: Meeting their Needs*. London: David Fulton, Chapter 4.

National Autistic Society (2001) *Approaches to Autism*. London: National Autistic Society.

Contact details for specific programmes in alphabetical order:

Art therapy

☎ 0044 (0)20 7383 3774   💻 www.baat.org

Auditory Integration Training (AIT)

☎ 0044 020 8880 1269   💻 www.light-and-sound.co.uk

Or,

☎ 0044 01273 474877   💻 www.listeningcentre.co.uk

Daily Life Therapy (Higashi)

☎ 001 617 961 0800   💻 www.musashino-higashi.org

Dance therapy

Contact: Association of Dance Movement Therapy, Bristol, BS3 5HX

☎ www.admt.org.uk

Early Bird (National Autistic Society)

☎ 0044 (0)1709 761 273   💻 E-mail: earlybird@dial.pipex.com

Lovaas

Parents for the Early Intervention of Autism in Children (PEACH)

☎ 0044 (0)1344 882248   💻 www.peach.org.uk

Makaton

☎ 0044 (0)1276 613 90   💻 www.makaton.org

Music therapy

☎ 0044 (0)20 8441 6226   🖥 www.bsmt.org

Picture Exchange Communication System (PECS)

☎ 0044 (0)1273 728 888   🖥 www.pecs-uk.com

Sensory integration

☎ 001 310 320 2335   🖥 www.sensoryint.com

Son-Rise (Options approach)

☎ 001 413 229 2100   🖥 www.option.org

Speech and language therapy

Advisers on Autism, Royal College of Speech and Language Therapists.

☎ 0044 (0) 020 7378 1200   🖥 www.rcslt.org

SPELL (National Autistic Society)

☎ 0044 (0)117 974 8400   🖥 www.nas.org.uk/schools

TEACCH

Treatment and Education of Autistic and Related Communication Handicapped Children

☎ 001 919 966 2173   🖥 www.teacch.com

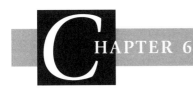

Providing for young children with autism

Introduction

Having explored definitions and characteristics of autism (Chapter 1), implications for families (Chapter 2), diagnosis and assessment (Chapter 3), the world of the child with autism (Chapter 4) and programmes of intervention (Chapter 5) this chapter will begin to pull together the threads and offer strategies for parents and practitioners. Key issues will be identified and discussed, and practical and realistic ideas for practitioners will emerge which will not only enhance practice, but also enable children with autism to participate more fully in the opportunities available to them. The case studies offered in Chapter 4 will be revisited to help clarify understanding.

Inclusion

In this era of inclusion in mainstream settings, more and more children with special needs, including those with autistic spectrum disorders, are now attending their local early years setting. This is further compounded by advances in medical science resulting in more children surviving conditions that may previously have resulted in early or premature death. Full inclusion would enable all children to attend their local mainstream setting with the staff of all settings having appropriate expertise, knowledge and skills to provide appropriately for their needs. This situation may be the ideal but in reality it is a situation we are still working towards in the UK. For continued positive progress, issues of funding, accessibility, training and resources will need to be addressed. In addition, the government will need to cease issuing legislation and guidance that is 'special needs' specific as, by doing so, special needs provision is segregated from 'normal' provision. Either we should aim to be inclusive or not.

For the child with autism we have a situation, for example, where parents may have researched widely and concluded that the Higashi approach is the most appropriate and therefore the desired option for their child. Their local authority may be unable to support this wish and despite increased levels of parental choice, this option may be denied them. A family in another area of the country may be supported by the LEA to initiate the Higashi programme or to fund attendance at a Higashi training programme. Thus equity of provision for children with autism is still an issue for improvement. Issues of inclusion will be further debated in Chapter 7.

Key areas of difficulty

The characteristics of autism discussed in chapters one and four gave us the three key areas of difficulty:

- social interaction;

- social communication;

- imagination.

These difficulties will often be accompanied by repetitive and stereotypical behaviours. If we are considering how best to accommodate these needs within our homes and early years settings, prior understanding and awareness of the features of autism and the resulting effects on the child, family and setting are essential. Unless we fully understand the difficulties experienced by the children we cannot begin to plan appropriate strategies to support the child's development and to enable greater participation.

Good practice for supporting children with autism

When discussing aspects of good practice in any early years setting practitioners need to be clear how they are measuring good practice and against which criteria. Early years settings need to satisfy OFSTED requirements and, therefore, output measures may be the guiding criteria to work with. It could be suggested, however, that for the individual child with autism the levels of performance on entry (baseline performance) and the amount of progress made as a result of the input of the setting are perhaps more realistic and child specific, which cannot always be equated with OFSTED requirements. Success with individual children and enabling greater participation could be judged as the most important measures of success and, therefore, indicative of good practice. Good practice by individual practitioners could be assessed according to their knowledge and understanding of autism, which leads to improved provision and, hopefully, greater progress for the child. This would, in my view, be preferable to assessing how far the child had progressed when compared with the areas of learning within the Early Learning Goals (QCA, 1999). As previously suggested practitioners who are inflexible and have little knowledge and understanding of autistic spectrum disorders may inadvertently compound the child's difficulties and clearly this should be avoided. As Powell and Jordan (1997) suggest: 'there are still numerous examples of where teachers, especially perhaps in mainstream, either do not fully appreciate the nature and extent of the child's difficulties or are unwilling (or perhaps unable) to alter their own approach to teaching to accommodate these difficulties' (p. 17). Powell and Jordan continue to emphasize that understanding of autism should be a key priority for all practitioners working with children with autism.

The recently published good practice guidance documents suggest the following key principles that 'should underpin all aspects of practice when providing for children with an ASD' which would be a useful guide for reflection by settings:

- knowledge and understanding of autistic spectrum disorders;

- early identification and intervention;

- policy and planning;

- family support and partnership;

- involvement of children;

- co-operation with other agencies;

- clear goals;

- monitoring, evaluation and research (DfES/DoH, 2002, p. 15–18).

The good practice guidance continues to identify the 'Pointers' and the 'Evidence/features to look for' that would be indicative of sound and effective practice. On closer inspection, however, whilst early years provision is included within the document, there appears a possible lack of awareness of the realities of working in the field of pre-school settings. The role of SENCOs in supporting children with autistic spectrum disorders is discussed, as is the need for an appropriate range of provision for all children with autism. In addition, the need for speech and language therapy is highlighted, along with the need for staff training. Funding is discussed but is related more to policies and transparency. Whilst these are all valid, the issues of funding, access to speech and language therapy services, equality of access to provision and equality of access to training are not directly addressed and one can only assume that the funding for such arrangements is in place by way of the EYDCPs in each authority. However, practitioners I meet on training sessions often report how difficult it is to access training and how self-funding groups cannot afford the fees charged. These are clearly issues that still need attention. At a recent training session I attended, out of 40 participants only two had seen the good practice guidance documents, so clearly the messages are not, as yet, getting through. It would be hoped that over time all practitioners could have access to appropriate training, through locally and nationally initiated programmes, that will enable them to identify the features of good practice and effective provision based on a firm understanding of autistic spectrum disorders.

Early intervention

The notion of early identification and intervention is widely supported (DfES/DoH, 2002; Powell and Jordan, 1997; Siegel, 1996) but, whilst many may raise concerns about the labelling of very young children, which I agree can have disadvantages, is it not preferable to consider the early identification of an ASD as informing subsequent provision? If a child is confirmed as having autism, then practitioners who understand autism can ensure that appropriate intervention strategies are put in place. Whilst waiting for a diagnosis, the resourceful and knowledgeable practitioner will already be implementing such strategies.

Early diagnosis will not necessarily lead immediately to appropriate interventions, as many parents have reported. They felt that a diagnosis should automatically lead to intervention but the reality was often very different, with long periods of time between the two stages and struggles to secure provision. Whilst some medical professionals or local authorities may prefer to delay diagnosis to enable further, more detailed, assessments of progress, research shows that earlier is certainly better for the young child with autism. Siegel (1996) concluded that:

> The earlier intervention starts, the better. What we do know is that most brain growth, and most fundamental aspects of learning, takes place in the first six years of life. This is really the prime time for intervention. You can think of it as a period of time when you can get in there and re-wire the circuits or re-write the software – and that the efforts will be more effective early rather than later. (p. 84)

Devising appropriate support

When devising appropriate support for a child with autism the practitioner will need to consider each child individually, as is good practice in any early years setting. The child's strengths and weaknesses will be a focus and the skilful use of the child's preferred resources and learning styles will be more likely to result in success. If this is combined with practitioner understanding of the particular difficulties experienced by the child and how best to respond to those difficulties, then the support will be more child specific and relevant. Each child with autism is different and it should always be remembered that what works for one child may have little positive impact on the next. The need for effective, flexible and resourceful practitioners is clear, but this should be accompanied with thorough training in the field of autism. One half-day 'Introduction to Autism' training session will not prepare practitioners adequately to provide for all children with autism who may arrive at their doors. It will simply begin their understanding of a very complex disorder. Any support staff that may work within the setting should also have relevant knowledge, or may inadvertently compound the child's difficulties resulting in possible confusion, fear and inappropriate behaviours.

Once the practitioner is working with the child, the setting itself should be adapted (where necessary) to support the child's activities and optimize learning potential. Individual education plans (IEPs) would be devised, monitored and reviewed regularly, and the Foundation Stage or National Curriculum will need to be used as a guide. Again, the skilful practitioner will not find it difficult to link the activities planned into the overall planning for the whole group. After all, the skills we aim to develop are the same as those for the other children in the group. The way we plan and prepare activities for individual children is the key.

In summary, appropriate support would involve:

- having knowledge and understanding of autism and being able to translate this into practice;

- making the learning environment supportive to the child with autism;

- devising meaningful IEPs that take into account strengths/weaknesses/likes/dislikes which are not based on a deficit model of remediation;

- implementing appropriate activities and teaching approaches.

- involving parents;

- incorporating regular observation, assessment and monitoring;

- using specialist expertise of outside professionals when needed;

- incorporating the Foundation Stage and/or National Curriculum;

- incorporating provision for the child with autism into overall planning;

- ensuring all staff, including support staff, have access to relevant training;

- support for family members.

It should always be remembered that we do not want simply to train young children to be able to perform set tasks in a robotic fashion, but to provide them with opportunities to develop their full potential in a meaningful way, enabling them to participate more fully in their environments. There is no set method nor range of strategies that will be appropriate for all children with autism, and the most effective practitioners will be unlikely to use only one approach or intervention programme. Many will take whichever elements or strategies are appropriate for each child and adapt them to be child specific. It may not be easy, as working with young children has always been a complex and highly skilled role, but the rewards can be plentiful. Progress may be slower than we would like, but as long as progress is consistent and ongoing then we should be satisfied.

Adaptations to the learning environment

From discussions in previous chapters we can conclude that children with autism need structure, routine, low distractibility and verbal cues to enable them more easily to function in an early years setting or home. For the learning environment this may require some basic changes.

The room should be structured with clearly defined areas indicated by written and/or pictorial signs. This offers clarity and security to the child and will reduce confusion and anxiety which could occur if a child does not know which area he/she is supposed to be in and what they are expected to do there.

Visual/written schedules or timetables for the child will indicate to the child which activities he/she should undertake and in which order. This will also offer clarity and routine once the child is able to use it. Confusion created by not knowing what will happen next, for how long and what may be asked of you, can be disconcerting for anyone, but is more pronounced in the child with autism.

For individual work or one-to-one teaching, a separate area with low distractibility and good access to any required resources is needed. This may mean that the practitioner needs to set up the resources and/or task prior to the session to enable the child to go to the work area and complete the task independently. Practitioners should remember that children with autism would need to know exactly what is expected of them, so if we want a child to thread six buttons on a lace then we only place six buttons and one lace in his/her tray or box. If we know the child likes red objects then it would be sensible initially to use only red buttons.

Strategies for developing social interaction

To develop a child's social interaction skills will involve providing activities to support the development of:

- interest in other people;
- tolerating the presence of other people;
- desiring interaction with others;
- eye contact;
- listening and attention skills;
- social play;
- turn-taking and sharing.

It should be remembered that to achieve all the above would take time, with progress being very slow at times. Any progress, however, should be celebrated no matter how slight. As long as each step is developmentally appropriate, and tasks have been broken down into small progressive steps, then success should follow. When trying to focus on one activity or stage, try to eliminate or reduce background noise and visual distractions to promote improved concentration.

Young children with autism may react very negatively to any attempts of social interaction or approaches from adults or children alike, resulting in head-banging, screaming, hand-flapping, covering eyes or ears. This is not unacceptable behaviour, but their way of coping with a situation they feel uncomfortable with or even fearful of. Use their preferred activity as a starting point to:

- imitate their actions nearby;
- reduce slightly the distance between you;
- talk about and develop your play a little – too much change may result in the opposite reaction;
- offer the child one of your toys;
- suggest the child makes a minor change to their set play routine, or, invite the child to join your game, or ask if you can join the child's game;
- praise any interaction shown.

The above staged process may be achieved within days or it may take weeks, but as long as development is evident, then time should not be a ruling factor. Once the child accepts the adult's presence and, hopefully, begins to watch and imitate the adult play model, then the beginnings of interaction are emerging.

Strategies to support social interaction skills could include:

1. Collecting your own toys for a simple imaginative game linked to the child's likes and preferred activities. Playing your game where the child can see you and displaying pleasure and enjoyment whilst describing and talking about your game. Inviting the child to join in or offer him/her one of the toys. The child may reject this invitation but if you repeat the exercise regularly he/she is likely to develop a desire to interact with you. This type of activity could include looking at and talking about a book.

2. Encouraging the child to participate in social activities such as storytime or snack time. Using a staged, progressive approach to the desired behaviour, beginning with the child's chair being apart from the group, facing another direction and next to their key worker's chair if his/her presence is acceptable to the child. The distance between the child and the group can gradually be reduced as progress is made. If the child's interest can be incorporated, then success may be more forthcoming.

3. Ensuring you indicate a desire to interact with the child through passing comments or smiling if he/she glances at you. Although the child may not initially show any interest in others, we should still show that we value and respect him/her.

4. If a child can tolerate your presence, try to encourage physical contact through stroking the child's arms or gently touching his/her shoulder to try to develop an awareness of touch as acceptable and even enjoyable. In time it may even be liked. (I can recall a little boy who developed a need for me to stroke his forearms when he was feeling under pressure or stressed. He appeared to be soothed and calmed by this action and would come to me, take my hands and place them on his fore-arms when in need of this support.)

5. Ensuring the child's safety due to the possible lack of aware-ness of danger and/or possible low sensitivity to pain. This can be achieved by placing visual barriers such as wide tape across dangerous items or, better still, having them cor-doned off and generally being aware of where the child is and what he/she is doing.

6. Eye-to-eye contact does not come naturally to all children with autism. If the child is approaching you, try to anticipate this and face him/her, give eye-to-eye contact and say 'hello' in acknowledgement, thus demonstrating the appropriate way to approach people. If the child will allow, tilt their head to directly face yours, even if they are glancing out of the corner of their eyes to avoid direct eye contact. Remember and respect that the child with autism may see eye-to-eye con-tact as difficult, challenging or possibly fearful.

7. Encouraging action rhymes by singing them to yourself if necessary, and performing the simple actions. If the child allows, move his/her hands to copy the actions. This not only develops imitation skills but interaction skills, attention and concentration, eye-to-eye contact, sharing and turn-taking.

8. Overemphasizing your facial or body gestures that are accompanied by verbal comment to support the develop-ment of understanding other people around you. You could also use pictures of facial expressions and match them, find a pair or just talk about them.

9. Drawing the child's attention to you before speaking to or interacting with him/her to signal that something will follow. By saying his/her name and pointing to your own eyes or ears will indicate to the child you want him/her to look or listen.

10. Continuing to show things to the child, despite the child not appearing to want to show you things. This will help develop an awareness of sharing, as well as helping to develop vocabulary.

11. Showing an interest and commenting on what the child is doing, even if it is a repetitive play routine. He/she may not be interested in you, but you should show an interest in him/her.

12. Rewarding any progress made by the child, either verbally and/or with a tangible reward. Even though the child may not initially understand the praise or what is being praised, this should develop in time. In addition, any child, with or without autism, is likely to repeat an activity or behaviour that is positively rewarded.

Strategies for developing social communication

Many children with autism will not progress through the expected stages of babbling and experimenting with their own vocal sounds. Most of us would agree that for young babies and children the motivation to communicate is very powerful, but for children with autism that innate desire, and thus motivation, is missing. Although we can see how beneficial it would be for a child with autism to communicate, the child may not see that need. This fundamental issue is of key importance when considering the development of communication skills. As some children with autism may be oversensitive to noise and background noise then activities should be planned to accommodate this. Perhaps the factor most influential for encouraging children with autism, is using resources and rewards that appeal to them. A basic human fact is that if we have a purpose or interest then we are more likely to want to participate.

It is essential that children with autism be provided with a means of communication and an ability to understand the communication of others around them. The rules of communication may not be readily understood by children with autism, but these can be developed through repeated modelling and imitation. If children do not develop verbal communication at a young age, this can be supplemented by introducing PECS or Makaton (see Chapter 5).

Some children with autism are able to develop a good level of social communication skills but some will remain with limited skills and predominantly non-verbal. To develop a child's social communication skills will involve providing activities to encourage:

- awareness of the basic ingredients of communication – eye contact, listening, concentrating, having people near to you and facing you;

- creating sounds and using the mouths for different purposes;

- pointing skills;

- strategies to indicate to an adult that he/she needs something (to move them on from taking you by the hand and leading you);

- object naming;

- early speech and language from one word utterances onwards;

- understanding meaning;

- understanding facial expressions and body language;

- understanding the meaning of short sentences as opposed to one or two words in the sentence;

- reducing echolalia (if used);

- understanding the rules and principles of communication.

Many of the preceding strategies for supporting social interaction, (numbered 1–12), will also be supportive of social communication development. In addition the following strategies can be useful:

1. When a child needs something:
   (a) encourage eye contact, perhaps by tilting his/her head;
   (b) face-to-face position;
   (c) encourage pointing to the object;
   (d) name the object within a simple sentence;
   (e) make a positive comment about the communication attempt itself and the object or activity you are being led to.

2. Encourage use of the child's name:
   (a) when the child approaches, greet him/her by name;
   (b) use the child's name when praising;

(c) call the child by name, even if you know he/she will not respond, then go to the child and repeat the name, encouraging eye contact and concentration;

(d) if the child can tolerate physical touch, when you call him/her, another adult could turn the child to face you and encourage a response.

3. When you speak to the child, always allow a short pause after, to allow the child to say or do something in return, just as in conversation.

4. When near to the child use simple language to describe what you are doing, so appropriate language models are heard.

5. Play games that involve turn-taking, sharing and making sounds, and using the mouth for a range of activities to encourage awareness of the mouth and sounds. Examples include blowing bubbles, making animal noises and sounds, blowing raspberries, swallowing, licking and making sounds at different pitches.

6. If the child makes unprompted sounds or noises, copy them to encourage further experimentation.

7. Make funny faces and different facial expressions, noises and sounds.

8. Use puppets to have conversations with. This will encourage understanding of the rules of conversation.

9. Talk about people's expressions in photographs, pictures and puzzles to encourage recognition and awareness of facial expressions, e.g. 'Daddy looks happy' or 'She's sad'.

10. Use rhymes, simple games and play to encourage taking turns and sharing. This will also help to develop an understanding of turn-taking in conversation.

11. Place labels (pictures and words) on objects around the room.

12. Repeat simple phrases often, and do not change them, e.g. 'Do you want a drink?'. This can be accompanied by an action, e.g. showing a cup.

13. Encourage the child to show you things, name them and talk about them in short, simple sentences. Be interested and

praise the action. Repeat the same simple phrase every time the object appears and touch it if you can, to relate the object to the word.

14. Link objects to actions to support understanding, e.g. when you say 'It's dinner time' hold up the child's fork or plate. Always use the same object.

15. Refrain from using confusing sayings, e.g. 'jump in the bath', when you actually mean 'get in the bath'.

16. Place pictures near objects you know the child may want, and encourage him/her to point to, or bring you, the picture, as opposed to just leading you to the area and you guessing what is wanted.

17. Place desired objects such as the child's cup, biscuits/crisps, favoured toys, just out of the child's reach to encourage the need for communication.

18. Have fun looking in a mirror, making faces and talking about your face. Give the child a second mirror so you can share the activity and encourage participation.

19. If the child attempts a word but gets it wrong e.g. 'gog' for dog, always offer the correct version – 'Yes, dog'.

20. Once the child has developed single-word naming, begin extension exercises by adding a word at a time to describe, e.g. 'Yes, a black dog'.

21. Use toys and objects to enact verbs, naming them at the same time, e.g. 'teddy is jumping'; 'teddy is sleeping'.

The above list is by no means exhaustive and practitioners and parents will be able to suggest many more activities to encourage and support the development of social communication skills.

Strategies for developing imaginative skills

Imagination and play are exciting and expected elements of the lives of young children. Seeing young children turn a cardboard box into a castle, charging around on broomstick 'horses', attempting to break into the castle and steal the queen is very rewarding. As adults we can all identify the wealth of learning that is underlying this fun activity. The child with autism is likely to play alone, resist interaction with others and repeat set play routines, such as lining up cars and driving them back and forth. The element of imagination and developing imaginative play is missing and the children do not have a need to develop these skills. The routine and structure of their play is comforting, reassuring and non-threatening as it excludes all other people. To begin development of imaginative skills practitioners and parents will need to work on:

- lack of imaginative play;
- rigid, repetitive or stereotypical behaviours;
- need for routine and structure and resistance to change;
- resistance to involvement in activities with others.

In line with other areas of development, progress is likely to be slow but consistent. If parents and practitioners can work together demonstrating consistency of approaches in both the home and the early years setting, this will offer security to the child. Using the child's preferred activities and capitalizing on strengths will also encourage positive progress. All those in contact with the child, including family members, any voluntary helpers or classroom assistants, will need to follow the same planned strategies. Strategies implemented to support the development of imaginative will include:

- routine and consistency;
- security for the child;
- flexibility;
- thorough and individualized planning;
- small progressive steps;
- use of imitation, modelling and verbalization;
- use of positive rewards;
- use of preferred toys and resources;
- realistic expectations;
- humour, enjoyment and excitement;
- adult involvement that encourages and rewards interaction from the child.

The importance of developing play skills

The use of play as a sound basis for establishing imaginative skills, as well as supporting social interaction and communication will be a key feature of planned activities. Recognition of the value of a play-based curriculum for the early years has been long awaited and the current Foundation Stage promotes play as a foundation for early learning. For young children, play usually begins with babies exploring objects around them through handling, sucking, mouthing and exploring them. Through this exploration of objects and the world around them, young children develop a whole range of skills including fine and gross motor, creative, mathematical, language and communication. When they confront a problem in their play they will try to solve it, sometimes through careful consideration and at other times through trial and error. All play-based learning is built on the foundations of prior learning, so by the age of 5 or 6 years young children are highly skilled individuals who can repeat play patterns, play simple games and demonstrate wonderful, exciting play routines. For the child with autism, the desire to explore the world and initiate interactions with people in their environment, is unlikely to exist, resulting in resisting interaction, lack of experimentation in play and resisting playing with others. Children with autism therefore need to be encouraged to play, shown how to play and how to expand their play routines, to enable further development and learning to take place. As Cumine, Leach and Stephenson (2000) state: 'It is, therefore, essential for practitioners to recognise that rather than teaching through play, play itself has to be taught to children with autism' (p. 67).

Through a staged approach, beginning with playing near the child with toys that are known to be appealing, parents and practitioners can first imitate the child's play routine to indicate support of his/her activity, but include verbal narrative of what he/she is doing. To demonstrate pleasure, enjoyment and excitement will be likely to arouse interest and should, hopefully, encourage the child's enjoyment. Over a period of time the adult can then extend the play a little to include additional moves and imaginative scenarios, again talking through the play as it develops. The child may then initiate interaction and add a toy to the adult's play, indicating interest and even desire to participate but not knowing how to go about it. If this happens, the adult will gently involve the child more and more over time. It may be that the adult sets up an identical play area, with the same toys for the child to use which are placed alongside the adult's. The child can then imitate the play modelled by the adult. With continued success the child will, hopefully, become more involved with the adult's play until they are both playing with the same set of toys in a parallel play situation. The final stages would be to move to co-operative play wherein both parties plan the next stage of the play routine with shared toys. If this kind of staged approach is used, it will offer security and confidence to the child and, hopefully, enable them to transfer the skills learnt in one play situation to another. Parents and practitioners, however, should be aware of the possibility that the child with autism may 'learn' the adult's play routine and simply repeat it as a set routine. The adult should persist with inviting the child to move the toys or perform his/her own next stage of the play routine to ensure that the child is bringing his/her own elements into the play, thus developing imaginative skills. More varied toys and routines can be added to maintain interest and to continue the extension of the child's play. Skills such as turn-taking and sharing will be used throughout the play sessions and adult narratives will encourage and support the development of communication, verbal or non-verbal.

As and when the child is considered ready, another child could be introduced into the planned play sessions to encourage interaction with another child. The 'new' child will more than likely support the play sessions in a natural way, through imitating, modelling, verbalizing, and, more generally, adding extra dimensions to the play situation. Over time it would be hoped that the adult could step back a little and leave the children to develop their own play sequences and, as long as positive progress is being made, the next stage should not be rushed for fear of undoing progress made.

Such staged approaches can also be used with stories, songs and rhymes, in the sand tray, water tray or home corner, in fact any focus can be used that is likely to appeal to the child. Knowledge of the child's strengths and weaknesses, likes and dislikes will inform the selection of play activities. Due to the child's preference for repetition it will be necessary to introduce changes gradually as, until the child becomes confident that the adult's play will be non threatening, he/she may react strongly and it could then be very difficult to resume the strategies without returning to the start.

Over time it would be hoped that the extension to the child's play routines and greater confidence in different play situations will help to reduce behaviours such as hand-flapping and head-banging that usually arise when the child is overly anxious, feeling threatened or uncertain of what is expected or what is happening and why. It is at these times that the child will be likely to resort to unusual body movements to cope with the 'difficult' situation, but through learning more useful, practical and enjoyable things to keep hands busy, the child is less likely to resort to unusual body movements.

Through careful planning, informed by observations of the child and discussions with parents, effective and staged play interventions will be supportive of the development of children with autism as summarized by Beyer and Gammeltoft (2000):

*Children with autism may benefit tremendously from play and we have been
astonished by the social competence shown by many of the children, when
they have been guided into the world of play. It is our responsibility to
design and set up an environment for these children based on their
particular needs in play. (p.14)*

To summarize, play routines will need to be carefully planned using a staged
approach to encourage positive outcomes. Each stage will be informed by
detailed knowledge of the child and results of prior observations, both formal
and informal. Progress may be rapid, slow or intermittent, but any observable
progress will be positive and rewarding.

Strategies for dealing with obsessive, repetitive and difficult behaviours

Difficult or repetitive behaviours can cause a range of problems as they can
manifest as temper tantrums, screaming (very loudly and for long periods),
slamming doors consistently, self-harming or harming others and/or poor
sleeping. These can occur at any time, continue for long periods of time and
often without much warning, at home, in public and/or the early years setting.
Clearly major difficulties can arise for families and practitioners, as they will
need to deal with these as appropriately as they can. Due to lack of public
awareness, and sometimes early years staff and parents, responsible adults
may feel intimidated by comments and negative feedback received from other
adults. Some parents have been asked to remove their children from their
local setting or a public place and onlookers may assume that the adults are
bad parents or carers.

Having explored the characteristics of autism and key areas of difficulty
we can now begin to appreciate the reasons for such outbursts, which could
be caused by:

- fear or confusion;
- anxiety;
- inability to communicate the source of the problem;
- over- or under-sensitivity;
- inability to cope with change;
- the need for structure, routine and 'sameness' in environments.

Identifying the cause of the difficulty will inform how it could be addressed. To begin addressing behaviours which are creating difficulties, parents and practitioners will need to identify exactly which behaviours need addressing and which of those would be the priority. Multiple behaviours cannot be dealt with all at once, so prioritization will be essential. Some of the strategies already offered in this chapter will be useful, but specific strategies that could be used to address behaviour difficulties and repetitive behaviours would include:

- always using positive rewards for any positive behaviours demonstrated;

- maintaining structure and routine as far as possible across all environments, e.g. having multiples of the favoured cup or even all crockery and cutlery, for use in all places – at home, setting or in public;

- keeping rules simple and clear, displayed in written and pictorial forms;

- using visual timetables to support understanding of what will happen next;

- using calming techniques that are known to work with the child, e.g. soft music, stroking;

- supporting the development of communication skills, verbal or non-verbal;

- sticking to set mealtimes and resisting giving the child snacks in between;

- acknowledging the child's over- or under-sensitivity and known fears;

- using visual clues whenever possible to support understanding;

- developing play and imaginative skills to divert attention to alternative and preferable activities;

- introducing activities gradually and preparing the child for expected changes;

- accommodating the child's likes/dislikes and preferred activities as far as possible, but without allowing domination by the child;

- incorporating the child's repetitive behaviours in a planned approach to extend skills;

■ limiting choices to avoid confusion;

■ using time out;

■ restricting repetitive or obsessional activities to set times only.

If one behaviour becomes more problematic, then a planned behavioural intervention may be implemented. This could incorporate:

■ defining the behaviour in observable terms. For example: 'He screams whenever the vacuum cleaner is used', is clear and observable, whilst 'He creates fuss, screams and is impossible', is too general;

■ observation and recording of the behaviour to identify specific facts and note any triggers or consequences;

■ consideration of all possible causal factors;

■ planning an individual intervention to address the behaviour;

■ implementing the intervention;

■ continued monitoring and observations to highlight progress (or otherwise);

■ evaluation of the process.

Linking with the Foundation Stage and the National Curriculum

Although some parents and practitioners may suggest that a child's difficulties are such that the Foundation Stage curriculum or National Curriculum would be inappropriate, on closer examination it should be realized that linking the planning for children with autism into a standard curriculum is not impossible. For children with autism greater emphasis will need to be placed on activities to support difficulties allied to the triad of impairments, but these activities, whilst having a strong focus, can be matched to the curriculum.

Illustrative example 6.1

Jason, aged 3, who was discussed in Chapter 4, demonstrated the following social interaction difficulties:

■ No desire to play with others.

■ Avoiding interaction with key worker.

■ Runs his train back and forth along the window ledge, but looks up when a rescue vehicle passes outside with the siren blaring.

■ Screams and places his hands over his ears if anyone takes his train away.

■ Resistant to alternative play activities.

■ Ignores snack and social times.

■ No verbal communication skills.

The setting implemented strategies similar to those outlined within this chapter, specifically to address Jason's social interaction difficulties. The key worker began imitating his play alongside him, talking about what she was doing, she introduced a fire engine to her play and placed another on the floor which Jason eventually took to incorporate in his play. Over a period of two weeks the key worker inched their play closer together and introduced a simple four-piece jigsaw of Fireman Sam, which she repeatedly completed. Again he decided in his own time that he wanted to explore this jigsaw. The system of support continued and expanded over a period of months and gradual progress was made. Areas of the Foundation Stage that could be linked with these strategies are given below and are coded thus:

■ Personal, social and emotional development – PSE

■ Communication, language and literacy – CLL

■ Mathematical development – MD

■ Knowledge and understanding of the world – KUW

■ Physical development – PD

■ Creative development – CD (QCA, 2000).

PSE: feeling safe, secure and able to trust the practitioner; learning to respect self and others; developing self-image; developing relationships; developing a positive disposition to learning; opportunities to problem-solve.

CLL: opportunities to develop speaking and listening and represent ideas; using communication and language; offering opportunities for communication.

MD: encouraging mathematical understanding of space, number, size etc.; opportunities to practise mathematical knowledge and understanding.

KUW: interaction with others; gathering information.

PD: opportunities to develop fine and gross motor skills; working in a safe environment; developing senses; promoting confidence and independence.

CD: feeling secure to try new experiences.

So, clearly, the activities individually planned for Jason can be linked to the Foundation Stage and Early Learning Goals (QCA, 1999; 2000). Similar strategies could be devised for Emma and James, who were also discussed in Chapter 4, which could also be linked to the areas of learning and Foundation Stage requirements. Individual education plans will indicate to parents and outside agencies that the selected activities are not only individually tailored to the child's needs but are closely linked to the Foundation Stage. This would also ensure that settings are able to demonstrate accountability.

Individual education plans

Within the Code of Practice (DfES, 2001b) any child with special needs who does not respond to initial interventions will be moved on to the graduated response stage of Early Years Action. Wall (2003a) summarizes the process: 'At this stage information will be collected from parents and other professionals involved with the child, and practitioners, along with the SENCO, will be in an informed position to suggest ways forward. Formalizing future plans will involve the creation of an IEP ...' (p. 116).

Individual education plans should offer clarity and precision to the individual planning and provision for children with autism, including the following information:

- name, birthdate and age of the child;
- specific difficulties experienced by the child;
- areas of the child's strengths;

- involved professionals;

- short-term targets;

- strategies to be used (including resources, staffing and interventions);

- parental views and involvement;

- monitoring and review plans and dates;

- exit criteria.

Any targets produced in an IEP should be realistic, time restricted, achievable and child specific. Whilst there is no set format for IEPs, they should be easy to read and understand, not too lengthy and readily accessible to parents and practitioners alike. As an ongoing working document an IEP will be a fundamental element of provision for children with autism.

Summary

Throughout this chapter features of good practice for providing for children with autism, along with a range of strategies for supporting individual needs, have been identified and explored. With a sound underpinning knowledge of autistic difficulties it is hoped that practitioners may be more confident to implement strategies that have taken into account the reasons for the child's difficulties, the effects on the child, family and setting and the implications of those difficulties. Working with all other professionals involved with the child, and having established an effective two-way partnership with parents, will further inform practitioners.

The issues of access to training, funding and resources (human and otherwise) will be critical to ensure appropriate provision for all young children with autism and these are ongoing issues. Yet, even if all early years practitioners were fully trained, as one child can be so different from another, the flexibility and resourcefulness of professionals will play a significant role. Selecting and implementing strategies which are individually tailored to the child's needs and close liaison between all staff and the child's parents will be most likely to secure progress. This would include some training for ancillary staff who will come into contact with the child regularly as their lack of understanding could counteract some of the skilful work of the practitioner.

Key issues

■ *Play-based approaches for children with autism will encourage the development of a range of skills.*

■ *Individual planning is essential and can be linked into whole group planning and the curriculum (Foundation Stage or National Curriculum).*

■ *Underpinning knowledge of autism is crucial for effective provision.*

■ *Flexibility and resourcefulness of practitioners will have a significant impact on responding to the individual needs of the children.*

Some suggestions for discussion

Item 1

Focus on a child with autism you are working with or have worked with in the past and list their strengths and weaknesses, likes/dislikes and difficulties in the area of social interaction and/or social communication. Begin to explore appropriate strategies that could be implemented.

Item 2

Repeat item 1 but reflect on the child's difficulties with imaginative skills and repetitive behaviours.

Item 3

Link the strategies you have developed in items 1 and 2 above to the Early Learning Goals or National Curriculum.

Item 4

Reflect on how you involve parents in planning, devising and implementing strategies. Does your current system allow them to use the same strategies outside of the setting and support them during the implementation stages to ensure consistency of approach? If not, how could this be addressed?

📖 Suggested further reading

Beyer, B. and Gammeltoft, L. (2000) *Autism and Play.* London: Jessica Kingsley.
Jordan, R. and Libby, S. (1997) 'Developing and using play in the curriculum', in S. Powell and R. Jordan (eds), *Autism and Learning: A Guide to Good Practice.* London: David Fulton, Chapter 3.

Leicestershire County Council and Fosse Health Trust (1998) *Autism – How to Help your Young Child.* London: National Autistic Society.

Seach, D. (1998) *Autistic Spectrum Disorder: Positive Approaches for Teaching Children with ASD.* London: NASEN, Chapter 5.

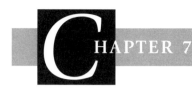

CHAPTER 7

Mainstream or special? Issues of inclusion

Introduction

I ssues of inclusion continue to be a focus for debate: inclusion in society, in the workplace, in the local community, in school and in early years settings. Within this chapter the history of educational inclusion will be presented to place later discussions in context. Combined with the knowledge of autism gained from previous chapters, practitioners should be placed in a more informed position to consider issues of inclusion within their own philosophy and relative to their early years setting.

Historically, early years providers have been accommodating of all children and have sought to provide the best for each and every child. However, is it realistic to expect practitioners to provide effectively and appropriately for the individual needs of *all* children? Do all practitioners have the relevant knowledge, expertise and skills? Is mainstream the most appropriate provision for every child with autism? Questions such as these will be explored within this chapter, highlighting the necessity for understanding and awareness of autism in order to provide appropriately. The concern that, for those with little or no understanding, more harm than good can in fact be done will again be emphasized.

Historical developments in inclusive education

Although a more detailed discussion of general historical developments can be found in Chapter 1 it is pertinent to review the key dates with more specific regard to children with autism and inclusive education.

The Education Act of 1944 (Ministry of Education, 1944) led to the appointment of a Minister for Education. Within the Act came the first clear acknowledgement that children with special needs should be considered separately, stating that: 'The Minister shall make regulations defining the several categories of pupils requiring special educational treatment and making provision as to the special methods appropriate for the education of pupils of each category' (ibid., p. 27). The Act continued to identify the need to provide for children with special educational needs in special schools if the 'disability is serious'. The following year the Handicapped Pupils and School Health Regulations (1945) identified the 11 categories to be used: blind, partially blind, deaf, partially deaf, delicate, diabetic, educationally subnormal, epileptic, maladjusted, physically handicapped and those with speech defects. At this stage all children with identified special needs were fitted into one of these categories and were subject to provision that was deemed appropriate for the disability. Autism was still in the very early stages of recognition and definition by Kanner, so was not considered within the categories of the 1945 Act.

The next significant legislation was the 1970 Education (Handicapped Children) Act (DES, 1970) placing responsibility and decision-making for children with disability into the hands of the Department of Education. As a result special schools developed, each with their own specialism and focus, such as severely subnormal, thus continuing the theme of separate, segregated provision.

The first national reference to early years special needs provision came within the Court Report of 1976 (Court, 1976). The report highlighted the need for greater focus on the screening of children in the early years to identify potential difficulties within a developmental framework.

In 1978 the Warnock Report (DES, 1978) reported on the review of provision for all 'handicapped children and young children' and Wall (2003a) suggests: 'This report, innovative at the time, was to inform subsequent legislation and significantly change the face of special educational needs' (p. 12). One of the key issues raised was that all children have a right to be educated and should be offered opportunities to support them in developing their full potential, which is indicative of society's view at that time in history. Another issue related to integration. Through a reflection of the provision at that time, three main forms of integration were identified within the report:

- locational – separate special provision on a school site. The children do not participate in mainstream activities;

- social – separate provision on a school site but with the children joining their mainstream peers for some sessions, e.g. art, music, lunch and play times;

■ functional – children are full-time participants in mainstream classrooms.

The following year the 1981 Education Act (DES, 1981) echoed the principles and recommendations of the Warnock Report. Within this key legislation definitions of special educational needs were clarified, formal assessments of special needs were introduced, categories of disability were removed with a greater focus on individual needs, parental partnerships were introduced and integration was to be encouraged. This was the first real move away from segregation for all children with special needs.

In 1993, part three of the Education Act (DfEE, 1993) addressed the difficulties that had evolved in the years since the 1981 Act. Guidance was offered on both the identification and assessment of special needs and SEN tribunals were created. This was followed in 1994 by the *Code of Practice* (DfEE, 1994) which offered detailed guidance on all aspects of special educational needs provision including:

■ identification of SEN;

■ assessment of SEN;

■ a five-staged assessment approach culminating in a statement of SEN;

■ regular reviews of progress, provision and statements;

■ introduction of the special educational needs co-ordinator (SENCO) (Wall, 2003a, p. 15).

The *Code of Practice* has subsequently been updated and revised (DfES, 2001b). Legislation and guidance have continued to emerge and there appears to have been a great increase in the arrival of successive documents, guidance booklets and legislation onto the desks of early years practitioners in all agencies. Each of these requires familiarization and implementation, so the requirements and expectations placed on practitioners have been considerable. The key documents (relating to early years, special needs and autism) include:

■ *Early Learning Goals* (QCA, 1999);

■ *Curriculum Guidance for the Foundation Stage* (QCA, 2000);

■ *Access to Education for Children and Young People with Medical Needs* (DfES, 2001a);

■ *Inclusive Schooling: Children with Special Educational Needs* (DfES, 2001a);

■ *Special Educational Needs Toolkit* (DfES, 2001c);

■ *Special Educational Needs and Disability Discrimination Act 2001* (DfES, 2001a);

■ *Autistic Spectrum Disorders: Good Practice Guidance* (DfES/DoH, 2002).

Definitions of inclusion

Everyone will already have his/her own personal understanding of the term 'inclusion' and definitions of inclusion will vary according to personal experiences and awareness of inclusion issues. In the widest sense inclusion within a society could be interpreted as allowing access to, and full participation in, all aspects of that society, for all people, at all times. Within the early years field, practitioners may narrow the focus down further and relate their definition specifically to local provision for young children. In this context inclusion could mean ensuring that all children have access at all times to the full range of activities and services available within the local community.

If such inclusive provision existed, then we would no longer be adapting buildings and planning separate activities for some of the children we work with, as the inclusive system would automatically accommodate the individual needs of all children. For the purposes of this chapter, inclusive early years provision for children with autism will be considered as *a process which enables young children with autism to be active participants in local early years settings, which removes all potential barriers to full inclusion in the range of opportunities offered. Such a process will account for individual needs and enable children to develop their full potential.*

It could be suggested that this definition relates directly to effective early years provision in a more general sense, but the key difference will be the knowledge, expertise and skills of the practitioners when providing for young children with autism. As has been expressed previously in this book, practitioners who do not have knowledge of autistic spectrum disorders and the resulting effects on the child combined with the implications for the setting, will be unlikely to be able to provide effectively for those children. Ignorance of autistic knowledge can lead to inappropriate activities which may compound the child's difficulties. The quality of the provision and skills of the practitioners are arguably much more important than the choice, or title, of setting itself.

Current provision for children with autism

Currently in the UK there is no standard form of provision for young children with autism. As with early years provision in general, provision for children with autism has emerged in response to greater numbers of children diagnosed with an autistic spectrum disorder and this has not necessarily developed in a coherent, thoroughly planned, manner. The result is a range of provision that is fragmented and does not support a fully inclusive system of provision. Provision in different areas will vary according to the knowledge and understanding of practitioners, access to appropriate training, the range of settings that can provide for children with autism, current legislation and the philosophy of the local authority at the time. From a parental perspective this may limit options and choice.

Parents will clearly understand the difficulties their child experiences better than anyone else and, if they have been well informed as to the range of approaches for providing for children with autism, they may have decided that a specific form of intervention would be best for their child. This may or may not be available within their own local authority. Further, the local authority may offer a place at a setting that the parents do not believe, for any number of reasons, will be able to provide effectively for their child. A whole range of issues emerges. Finding the right setting for your child can thus be problematic for parents of young children with autism. When this is considered alongside the range of other difficulties parents of children with autism can face, this could be suggested as yet another obstacle to their lives which should be resolved, at national and local levels, as soon as possible. The range of provision currently available includes the following placements.

1 Special schools specifically for children with autism

Perhaps the biggest advantage of this type of provision is the specialist knowledge and expertise of the staff in providing for children with autism. With autism-specific training as an ongoing aspect of professional development, such staff should be the most highly skilled practitioners in their field. Based within a firm understanding of the effects and implications of autistic-spectrum disorders, the curriculum and allied individual activities would be tailor-made to suit the needs of the children, ensuring progression and success within a secure and safe environment that directly responds to the needs of children with autism.

Within the UK, the National Autistic Society runs its own schools and centres for children and adults with autistic spectrum disorders. In addition the NAS (1998) devised an accreditation scheme which is 'a highly specialised quality assurance and review service for schools, units and classes catering for people with autistic spectrum disorders. The programme focuses on those key features which affect the suitability of placements for children with autism and provides a "seal of quality" from the National Autistic Society' (p. 2).

A range of settings specifically for children with autism clearly exists, with accreditation to the NAS but, again, availability will vary in different areas of the country. It may not be possible for all children to attend such a setting if their parents wished it. In many cases the fees would be paid by the local authority and without a diagnosis of autism, which as we have discussed can be delayed for a variety of reasons, attendance at such a setting may not be possible from an early age. In the interim period a child would probably attend a more local setting, either mainstream or special, which may, or may not, be able to provide effectively for their needs.

A further key benefit of autism-specific provision is that the whole ethos of the setting will revolve around appropriate organization and supportive features for the children. Daily routines, structure and visual clues would be evident throughout the setting and not just within the classrooms or activity rooms but also the dining halls, play and recreation areas, residential quarters (if residential) and administrative areas. This would offer reassurance, comfort and security to the children, thus enabling them to participate more freely and experience greater independence and control.

Segregated units do, however, by their very nature, separate children from the rest of the community and specifically, their local community and friends. It could be suggested that transfer back to mainstream provision could be more difficult when moving from an autism-supportive environment that truly understands the difficulties a child with autism would face. This period of transition is crucial and should be thoroughly planned with a system of gradual transition.

A potential difficulty with privately run provision is that without adequate monitoring and inspection processes the quality of the provision may be inappropriate, either in it's entirety or in part, which could have a negative effect on the children themselves and could lead to regression as opposed to progression.

There are, however, many highly successful schools for children with autism offering a broad curriculum, within small classes, supported by a range of interagency professionals and working closely with parents and the local community, that are enabling children to lead more independent lives and to make full use of the opportunities (educational and otherwise) offered to them. For these reasons, such a setting may be selected by parents as the most appropriate for their child, as they consider the provision might offer their child the best educational opportunities that are available.

2 Units attached to schools

A less segregated form of provision for children with autism would be a unit based on a school or community site, which offers the children autism-specific opportunities. Inclusion within the main school (whether it be a special school or mainstream) could occur at a range of levels from occasional visits to participation in everyday class activities some of the time. However, such inclusion must be managed effectively to ensure the appropriateness for individual children.

Benefits of such units would be the specific knowledge and skills of the unit staff and, therefore, the opportunities offered to the children, the provision being in the local neighbourhood and the opportunities to mix with their local peers within the main school. Clearly, if parents were offered, or are considering such a setting, they would need to visit and assess for themselves the appropriateness of the provision for their own child. If inclusion with the children from the main school is a key feature for parents they would need to assess the levels of such inclusion. The relevant knowledge and training of the unit staff may also be an area for investigation. Parents should not rely on the school prospectus alone but should make their own decisions and ask their own questions for clarity and to inform subsequent decisions. This does not relate solely to parents of children with autism seeking an appropriate setting, but would equally apply to any parent seeking provision of any sort for their child. We are all aware that establishments, whether academic or otherwise, can state they have policies for equal opportunities, but unless we see them for ourselves and question how they are translated into practice, there are no guarantees. As provision for children with autism is crucial, parents need to feel confident about their decisions regarding placements for their child.

3 Special schools

Special schools for young children could accommodate a range of disabilities including mild or severe learning difficulties, emotional and behavioural difficulties, specific disorders such as Down's syndrome and cerebral palsy, as well as complex difficulties. For this reason the staff would need to be knowledgeable in the wide range of disabilities for which they provide and ensure that provision is appropriate to individual needs.

Usually offering small classes, the adult:child ratio is likely to be highly favourable which maximizes opportunity, but problems could arise with whole-group activities due to the specific difficulties of children with autism. Although significantly impaired in social skills, some children with autism will demonstrate cognitive skills that are age appropriate or even in advance of their age. Similarly, the lack of social skills of the child with autism will mean highly skilled provision to support progress and to ensure the child is protected from any possible issues of intimidation or bullying by other children.

There are some very successful special schools providing appropriately for young children with autism but as with any provision, there are those whose provision could create a potential cause for concern. Invariably, the staff employed will be dedicated and highly skilled practitioners but they may lack autism-specific knowledge and expertise, which in turn could compound the difficulties of the children. As Howlin (1998) concluded: 'some schools for children with mild learning disabilities, or emotional and behavioural disturbance, can, and do, offer an effective educational environment. Unfortunately, in other cases, such provision may prove, at best, inadequate, and, at worst, psychologically or even physically harmful' (p. 242). Again it would be pertinent for parents to visit such schools which may be suggested as appropriate for their child and ask their own questions to ascertain the appropriateness of provision for the individual needs of their child.

4 Mainstream schools and early years settings

Increasingly, children with autistic spectrum disorders are placed in their local, neighbourhood settings. Whilst such inclusive practices are to be supported and commended, the quality and appropriateness of provision should be carefully considered with the individual child, in mind. Whilst such provision may be able to accommodate the needs of one child it could be highly inappropriate for another. Individual decisions would therefore be essential.

For children at the more able end of the autistic spectrum, inclusion within local mainstream schools can be highly successful as long as staff are adequately trained and knowledgeable in issues relating to autism. Flexibility to differentiate the curriculum and alter day-to-day routines may also be necessary. However, considerable benefits can be experienced by the other children in the group or class and the wider setting, as well as the children with autism. With careful planning practitioners can encourage a supportive network amongst the children that will enable them to grow up with an increased acceptance of difference, whether it be autism, ethnicity or any other issue.

It would be hoped that increased inclusion across the range of mainstream provision would be supported by increased training, knowledge and expertise, to ensure that all children benefit from the mainstream experience. This would reduce the current situation in which some children with autism may do well in mainstream provision whilst others fare less well. It is inappropriate to move forward on the principle that, with luck, the child with autism will happen to meet a practitioner who understands autism and the implications that go with it, and is able to provide effectively for the child's needs. All children with autism should be assured provision by highly skilled and knowledgeable practitioners who understand the child's difficulties and provide opportunities to support the child's progress in all areas.

5 Other forms of placement

- Assessment centres – short-term placements to undertake detailed assessment of individual needs and thus inform longer-term placement decisions.

- Home based programmes such as Portage or the Lovaas approach providing for young children with autism.

With such a varying range of provision, decisions for parents can be confusing and are sometimes hampered by lack of available information and guidance. For parents with an effective relationship with their key professional there is a likelihood that they will not only seek advice, but also follow it. The informed practitioner would ensure that parents are offered all the information available relating to the range of options open to them, supplemented by introductions and visits.

The availability of provision will largely depend on where you live in the country and what is available in your area. The openness of the local authority and speed of diagnosis will also affect decisions. Whilst legislation supports parental choice of educational setting local authorities may have limited resources (human, physical and financial) to offer the type of setting the parents request. Limited funding may result in the parents being refused financial support at a school outside the authority's boundaries. At a time when many parents are vulnerable and under considerable pressure and strains, a battle over a placement can only have negative effects.

The Evans et al. report (2001), which explored and analysed local authority provision for children with autistic spectrum disorders, offers much information regarding the range and availability of appropriate provision. With regard to the range of provision available the report concluded that:

> ...placement in a particular provision was related more to local circumstances and availability than to an exact match between children's needs and what was on offer. However, placement was less of an issue than expertise: children with similar levels of difficulty can thrive and make progress in a range of different provision, both integrated and segregated. One of the key issues for parents was the level of training and experience in autism of the people working with their children. (Ibid., p. 80)

Such a statement supports previous discussions within this chapter. Within the report was an indication that the number of settings able to provide for young children with autism has increased considerably over the past 20 years, however, the number of places available still falls very short of prevalence figures, indicating that a large proportion of children with autism may not be in appropriate placements. These findings are supported by the research findings offered by Jones (2002) who highlighted that in 1988 only 29 per cent of local authorities offered provision for children with autistic spectrum disorders. This compares with 60 per cent of authorities in the figures for the year 2000. It should be noted, however, that due to changes in local authority structures the number of authorities has increased, thus affecting the results. Whilst the number of placements has increased, it should also be remembered that this alone does not guarantee the appropriateness of any individual provision.

The recent NAS survey of members prepared by Barnard, Prior and Potter (2000) highlighted that most parents were satisfied with early years provision but that as the children progressed through the statutory education system, levels of satisfaction decreased significantly. This clearly raises crucial issues. Another key issue raised indicated the concerning lack of knowledge of practitioners: 'Parents need more choice – very few schools have staff who are adequately trained and can provide the right level of support for children with autism and Asperger syndrome, and autism-specific provision is very limited. Some young children have to travel long distances' (ibid., p. 7). This is also highlighted later in the same report when it is stated that 20 per cent of children with autistic spectrum disorders are excluded from their setting at some stage during their attendance. The report suggests that this was 'quite frequently because of a lack of staff with autism experience' (ibid., p. 8). So, yet again, the issue of appropriate levels of practitioner training, knowledge and experience is highlighted.

Issues of inclusion

It has emerged throughout this chapter that provision for children with autism varies across the country and a range of inclusion issues surface because of this. Different forms of provision will have strengths and weaknesses, and the suitability for individual children cannot be generalized. The levels of training, expertise, knowledge and skills of the practitioners are more important than the physical nature of the setting or whether it is a mainstream or special setting. Effective provision for young children with autism can only be successfully implemented by knowledgeable practitioners. Further, those that do not have appropriate and up-to-date training are unlikely to be able to provide effectively and may inadvertently compound the child's experiences, causing the child confusion, uncertainty and an inability to benefit from the opportunities available.

Availability of local, appropriate provision varies greatly and, therefore, affects parents' freedom of choice regarding a preferred placement for their child. The views and wishes of parents are fundamental to appropriate provision, as they know their child best. Family issues may affect their preferred placement and parents may have strong reasons for a specific choice. Having possibly reached this decision over time, to then be presented with obstacles at local authority level is compounding their difficulties further. This issue extends to areas of funding and authority budgets as the availability of provision will clearly be affected by access to appropriate levels of funding and support.

Levels of inclusion within settings will also vary greatly and whilst full inclusion and participation is to be encouraged and developed, it should be implemented within a supportive framework that accounts for the individual needs of young children with autism.

It could also be suggested that the move towards greater inclusion, whilst a commendable move in the right direction, has been implemented rapidly and that practitioners have had insufficient time to acquire appropriate levels of knowledge to ensure the effectiveness of such a process. The inclusion of children with autism should be carefully planned, implemented and monitored at national and local authority levels to ensure the quality of provision. Current special needs legislation and guidance, incorporating early years settings, has also been introduced very rapidly and has not necessarily resulted in improved provision. At a recent special needs training day in which I was involved, only one other person was aware of the good practice guidance documents released by the DfES/DoH in 2002. The lady also disclosed that she had only discovered the documents by accident when looking for another document on the Internet. This clearly raises an issue of consistency, as all those responsible for providing for children with autism should be familiar with all current legislation and guidance.

If inclusion aims to remove barriers of segregation, then the continued publication of guidance and legislation for children with autism, or any special need, should be discouraged. Whilst separate documentation continues to be produced, the notion of autism as a separate and discrete condition outside of the norm will persist.

Indications are that provision in the early years for children with autism is more successful than provision at later stages of education and this should be celebrated. The key features of good early years practice are also those of effective provision for children with autism. These features of good practice, however, will depend on the basic underpinning knowledge of autism and the effects and implications of all autistic spectrum disorders on the child, the family and the setting. Flexibility and understanding are crucial factors indicative of good practice.

Summary

Some general issues of inclusion have been offered within this chapter but the focus has been on inclusion for children with autistic spectrum disorders. Effective provision for young children with autism can occur in a range of settings that incorporate varying levels of inclusion. The government is currently driving towards increased inclusion, which most people would wholeheartedly support, however, any process of inclusion should be carefully planned, implemented and monitored to ensure effectiveness. The speed at which changes in special educational needs legislation and guidance have been implemented may be a cause for concern. Whilst such documentation clearly indicates the need for the appropriate training of practitioners and the rights of parents in decision-making, issues of the availability and access to the appropriate training have not yet been fully addressed. Parental choice of setting for their child cannot always be accommodated and the range of settings will vary according to geographical location. In addition, issues of funding and resources are not yet fully resolved. Not all early years practitioners have a sound underpinning knowledge of the effects and implications of autism, and it is only after this knowledge has been gained that practitioners can translate it into effective practice.

Emerging issues relating to inclusion and provision for children with autism would include:

- access to and availability of appropriate autism-specific training for *all* early years practitioners;

- speed of change in the fields of special needs and inclusive practices;

- funding;

- access to local provision for children with autistic spectrum disorders;

- the strengths and weaknesses of different approaches to inclusion for children with autism;

- knowledge and understanding of autism as crucial for effective provision;

■ inclusion should progress in a planned, developmental manner and cannot be rushed, as it is a process of change which cannot be achieved in the short term.

Unless inclusive practices can ensure that all children with autism will have their needs met effectively by highly skilled and experienced practitioners who have a sound knowledge of autistic spectrum disorders, then the difficulties of some children can, and will, be compounded inadvertently. Increased inclusion is to be commended but should not be rushed. Barnard et al.'s report (2000) significantly concludes that: 'If inclusion is not just an empty slogan it will require an effort' (p. 12). It could, therefore, follow that with increased commitment at national and local authority level practitioners could be supported to offer effective and inclusive practices to all young children with autistic spectrum disorders.

Key issues

■ Issues and barriers relating to issues of inclusion must be confronted and addressed to support future inclusive developments.

■ Access to a wide range of appropriate provision should be open to all families of children with autism.

■ All practitioners working with young children must be appropriately trained.

■ All children with autism are very different, just as all children are, and appropriateness of inclusive practices must be considered on an individual basis.

Some suggestions for discussion

Item 1
Compile a list of all settings in your local area that provide for young children with autism, and try to identify inclusive features of each.

Item 2
Consider the individual needs of a child with autism you are currently providing for. Reflect on the future placement of that child and identify which individual factors will need to be addressed to ensure the effectiveness of that provision for that child.

▶

▶

Item 3

Reflect on the inclusive practices of your own setting. As a staff discuss the strengths and weaknesses of those practices and identify any areas for possible improvement.

Item 4

In the light of your responses to item 3, identify ways to secure such improvements.

📖 Suggested further reading

Barnard, J., Prior, A. and Potter, D. (2000) *Inclusion and Autism: Is It Working?* London: NAS.

Jones, G. (2002) *Educational Provision for Children with Autism and Asperger Syndrome: Meeting their Needs.* London: David Fulton, Chapter 3.

National Foundation for Educational Research (2001) *Making a Difference: Early Interventions for Children with Autistic Spectrum Disorders.* Slough: NfER.

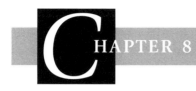

CHAPTER 8

Issues for consideration and suggestions for the future

Whilst developing themes throughout this book I have realized that I have barely scraped the surface of issues relating to provision for young children with autism. During my own working experiences I discovered barriers, both real and perceived, to my attempts to ensure the most appropriate and effective provision that I could offer. This, I learnt, depended to a great extent on my own understanding of the difficulties experienced by the children themselves and their families, and the resulting implications for the early years setting. On welcoming the first child diagnosed with autism into my setting I realized very quickly that my own knowledge was, to say the least, very limited. The 3-year-old responded to my attempts to interact, with screams, by covering his ears and stamping his feet, until I backed away. I had little idea of how to begin the process of establishing any form of communication and interaction with him. Without the basic knowledge of the characteristics of autism, the effects of autism and the implications for him, myself and the setting, I could not begin to attempt to provide appropriate activities. At the same time I was determined that the child received just as much attention and input as any other child that I worked with and that he should be provided with the opportunities to achieve his full potential.

My solution was to extend my knowledge as quickly as possible, which was achieved through attendance at seminars, training sessions and conferences combined with reading anything and everything I could find relating to autism, which I soon discovered was a considerable amount. Securing funding for these activities was an instant barrier, but this was not insurmountable. This little boy had equal rights to appropriate opportunities and I wanted to make sure they would be available to him. At that stage in time, children with autism were placed in special schools and nurseries, not mainstream, but today we are witnessing increasing inclusion into mainstream settings, which raises many issues if we are striving to meet the individual needs of all children with autism in our settings. It is hoped that this book will have supported and extended current levels of knowledge relating to autism, whilst at the same time reinforcing and celebrating existing good practice. When increased knowledge is combined with the expertise and skills of highly trained professionals, from whichever discipline, it is hoped that provision overall will be enhanced and the transition for children from the sometimes isolating world of autism into increased mainstream life will be made easier. Whilst autism is a lifelong developmental disorder, the skills of children with autism can be developed considerably to enable them to participate as more active members of their families, peer group and local community which will help them to achieve their own full potential, at whatever level that may be.

Crucial issues

Several key issues have emerged consistently throughout the chapters of this book, each of which is interlinked with the others. The first issue to consider is that of *diagnosis and assessment*. In Chapter 3 the difficulties of securing a definitive diagnosis of autism were highlighted, with experiences of families and research evidence informing the discussion. The problems of coping with a young child with autism were raised in Chapter 2 and clearly show that when children become 2 or 3 years of age their unusual behaviours can present a range of difficulties for other family members. The result can be that social circles are reduced or disappear and family life takes an unexpected, and sometimes difficult, direction. If problems arise when trying to secure a diagnosis, which should theoretically lead to appropriate provision, the family's difficulties are compounded further. It would seem that consistency of diagnostic approach should be an important issue for response at national levels. If all young children with autism were given an early diagnosis, following a thorough, multidisciplinary assessment, then the first step on the ladder may be made a little easier. Time lapses should be avoided as far as possible.

When future provision is considered for a child there should be a clear, national policy for *inclusion*, or segregation, depending on the child's individual needs, the family's preferred choices and the ability of local settings to provide appropriately. The government's drive for increased inclusion, whilst to be commended in principle, has been established very rapidly with legislation and guidance documents appearing regularly over recent years for practitioners to respond to. Changes in working practices have been required that have placed considerable pressures on already pressurized professionals. In addition, not all practitioners appear aware of all the latest documentation, including the recent *Autistic Spectrum Disorders: Good Practice Guidance*,

(OfES/DoH, 2002), which confirms that despite governmental support for those practitioners working with children with autism, the information is not reaching those who need it.

The whole inclusion debate also requires further clarity at national level, as currently the government is supporting inclusion, yet is still producing separate documentation for special educational needs, including documentation relating to autism. In addition, documentation clearly identifies that for some children separate special provision will still be needed. This presents a contradiction, as simply through producing separate documentation the government is sending out a message of inclusion for the majority but segregation for a minority, whilst at the same time continuing to expect increased inclusion.

The next issue concerns *access to appropriate and effective provision*, in every locality, for all children with autism whose parents desire it. This could be a range of special and mainstream provision. We have seen in previous chapters that the diversity of early years provision across the country currently varies considerably, with some areas offering a variety of approaches to autism that are accessible to all parents wherever they live, whilst others offer little choice. This situation has evolved on a needs-led, local basis, so overall there is a lack of consistency, and thus equity, for children and families. The result means that when parents have secured a diagnosis of autism, with all the difficulties that can involve, they can then be faced with another battle to secure preferred and appropriate provision. This issue can also be linked to *funding*, as funding may be cited as the reason for the lack of a range of provision in the local area, or the lack of availability of adequate funds to allow parents to secure attendance at a preferred centre out of the county.

If local mainstream provision is preferred by the parents, and/or encouraged by the local authority, it may be that the local provider cannot offer the expertise and knowledge required to ensure effective provision for the child. Inadvertently, an otherwise experienced practitioner who is not fully aware of the issues of autism can do more harm than good, despite having the best of intentions.

This then leads onto the issue of *training*. It could be suggested that within a system of inclusive provision all early years practitioners should have up-to-date and ongoing training in all areas of special needs provision, including autism, to ensure the effectiveness of the services they offer. To ensure this, a national network of training initiatives would be needed, led by the government, with support and guidance from appropriate bodies, organizations and parents. Then all practitioners would be equipped with the basic knowledge to inform working practices, thus ensuring effective provision for children with autism. This would also mean that more children with autism could be placed in their local settings, which would have the additional benefit of encouraging increased public awareness and understanding of autism.

Currently, access to appropriate training for early years practitioners varies considerably according to geographical location and access to funding to pay for the training, which highlights a related issue of equity. In my own experiences I have found that training days are mostly attended by early years teachers who are funded by their schools, whereas practitioners from settings such as pre-school groups and day nurseries, who are less likely to be funded, do not attend in great numbers. In addition, those from pre-school settings often struggle to find cover in the absence of the practitioner. This issue could be taken up at local authority level, via the Early Years Development and Childcare Partnerships, as well as nationally, to ensure increased participation in appropriate training.

Small-scale research project

The need for and access to appropriate autism related training has been an area of concern for me for a considerable time and to this end I recently conducted a small-scale research project to explore further issues of access to training for early years practitioners. Questionnaires were sent to 580 early years settings in the south of one county in England. The return rate was surprisingly high with 183 completed questionnaires being returned (31.55 per cent). Whilst the data is yet to be fully analysed, responses to key questions have been examined and support the current discussion within this chapter. The responses according to settings can be seen in Table 8.1, indicating responses from 97 primary school staff, 50 pre-school group staff, 27 private day nursery staff, 5 private nursery school staff, 3 playschemes/out-of-school club staff and 1 state day nursery staff member. In total, 12 males responded with the remaining 171 being female, reflecting the lack of male staff in early years settings.

Table 8.1 Responses according to settings

Type of setting	Number
Pre-school groups	50
Private nursery schools	5
Private day nurseries	27
State day nurseries	1
Primary schools	97
Playscheme/out-of-school clubs	3
Total	183

Table 8.2 Autism training undertaken in the last five years

Type of setting	0	1	2	3	4	5+	Total
Pre-school groups	40	8	0	0	0	2	50
Private nursery schools	3	2					5
Private day nurseries	23	3	1				27
State day nurseries	1						1
Primary schools	28	30	15	3	2	19	97
Playscheme/out-of-school clubs	2	1					3
Total	97	44	16	3	2	21	183

On asking for a list of any autism training undertaken in the last five years the responses offered me no surprises (see Table 8.2). In total, 97 practitioners (N = 183) had had no training, but 86 had undertaken some training. The emphasis must rest with the fact that the preliminary findings suggest that just over half have not undergone autism-specific training.

When practitioner training is further matched to setting type, more significant information emerges. Namely that 71.13 per cent of primary school practitioners have had at least one autism training session in the last five years, as opposed to only 20 per cent of pre-school practitioners. This is indicative of supporting evidence to my proposition that primary school staff would be more likely to be funded, and therefore attend, training, and thus equity of access to training is an emerging and vital issue.

Table 8.3 Practioners who would like to undertake autism training during the next academic year

Type of setting	Yes		No		Total
Pre-school groups	39	(78%)	11	(22%)	50
Private nursery schools	4	(80%)	1	(20%)	5
Private day nurseries	24	(89%)	3	(11%)	27
State day nurseries	1	(100%)	0	(0%)	1
Primary schools	50	(52%)	47	(48%)	97
Playscheme/out-of-school clubs	2	(67%)	1	(33%)	3
Totals	120	(66%)	63	(34%)	183

When asking if practitioners would like to undertake autism training during the next academic year the results were a clear indication of the desire for appropriate training (see Table 8.3). This issue should not pass without reflection if we are striving to support practitioners, and thus the children they work with, on a daily basis.

Due to the small-scale nature of this project, and the fact that only pre-liminary figures and findings were available at the current time of writing, generalizations and grand claims cannot be made, but the evidence is suffi-cient to highlight a situation which warrants further and more intensive study. It is hoped that the project will be written up and published in appropriate academic journals for interested parties to further explore the outcomes. However, for the purposes of this chapter, the preliminary results are a clear indication in one area of the country that early years practitioners, and partic-ularly those in pre-school settings, not only have a lack of training in autism, but are also eager to improve their knowledge and thus their effectiveness as providers for young children with autism. It could be suggested that this requires addressing as a matter of urgency.

Further key issues

Within Chapter 1 the development of early years provision was discussed alongside developments in legislation relating to special needs. This provided the background information regarding developments to date which is required to understand the current situation relating to legislation, guidance and provision. Definitions of, and developments in, the field of autism were also given to support increased understanding and to highlight the impor-tance of understanding the characteristics of autism within the triad of impairments. Without this fundamental knowledge it could be suggested that practitioners cannot truly begin to respond to the needs of the young child with autism. With diagnoses of autistic spectrum disorders increasing, com-bined with the ongoing movement towards greater inclusion, mainstream settings are increasingly expected to accept children with special needs in gen-eral, but also more children on the autistic spectrum. If practitioners do not have the underpinning knowledge of autism and the effects on all involved, then appropriate provision cannot be guaranteed. When the preliminary find-ings of the small-scale research project are combined with the above issue regarding training, then clearly a need to address the issue is identified.

Discussion in Chapter 1 also identified features of good practice in pro-viding for children with autism, which demonstrates similarities with effective early years practice. It could be suggested that effective early years practitioners will have the expertise, knowledge and skills to provide for children with autism providing they have the underpinning knowledge of autism. The issues concerned with the increased inclusion of young children with autism were also explored within the context of the ever-increasing legislation and guidance that emerges from government and national bodies. The main concern is that many early years practitioners work part-time hours for very limited financial reward and, therefore, expectations of this magnitude are considerable and perhaps unreasonable. However, as early years settings are subject to OFSTED regulations then these are firm requirements for practitioners and the settings in which they work.

Chapter 2 explored the specific issues relating to families of children with autism. Within current legislation and guidance the rights of parents are now considerable and early years practitioners need to be clear on the importance of this area of their work. The following question raises the profile of this particular area, 'Considerable time is spent in planning for children with special needs, but do we consider the needs of their families?' (Wall, 2003b, p. 62). The influences of family members on any child are well documented (Barnes, 1995; Wall, 2003a) and the effects of having a child with special needs and/or autism in the family are similarly well documented (Carpenter, 1997; Dale 1996, Harris 1994, Wall, 2003a). If we accept that families have a significant effect on the children, and vice versa, then practitioners cannot overlook the importance of this area. Government requirements have raised the profile and rights of parents regarding their children's education over recent years, and parent partnership schemes now exist within all local authorities. In addition, a wide range of parent-run groups and charities have emerged to campaign for the rights of parents of children with special needs. One of the key issues raised within Chapter 2 was the need for understanding individually the perspectives of mothers, fathers, siblings and grandparents. Once practitioners begin to reflect on the differing needs of parents of children with special needs they will be better placed to support family members more effectively.

A critical time for parents was that of diagnosis, and the need for specially trained, sensitive and discrete professionals to support them at this time was identified, as this would set the tone for future parent and professional contact. Access to relevant and up-to-date information was seen as essential by parents. In general, parents needed professionals to understand the difficulties they were experiencing in their everyday lives and the impact the child with autism was already making on the family, which could result in considerable pressure on all family members. If the complexities of the current situation could be appreciated then perhaps greater sensitivity could be demonstrated at the time of diagnosis. Parental reactions to diagnoses can vary greatly, from relief at knowing, to complete denial. Some parents appear to deal with the impact of diagnosis quickly and effectively, moving on almost instantly to the next stage in the process, whilst for others much more time will be needed.

However parents manage this difficult situation, the professionals involved need sensitivity, above all else. As well as the diagnosing professional, the practitioners within the early years setting will need to be sensitive and supportive to the parents at this time. As the professionals in most regular contact with the parents it is commonly the early years setting that will cope with an array of questions, problems, issues and the emotions, and feelings of the parents at the pre- and post-diagnosis stages.

To support family members effectively early years practitioners should be familiar with the range of supporting agencies in the local area so that parents can be introduced to groups that may be able to offer more specific support. Practitioners' existing knowledge of individual family members should inform effective support.

Illustrative example 8.1

Jenny and Richard have a 3-year-old son, Thomas. Thomas, like his two older sisters, was developing along expected developmental pathways until he reached his second birthday. After that, the vocabulary he had developed gradually disappeared, until he reached a stage when he no longer communicated verbally. During the same period he changed from a mischievous toddler who was interested in everything and everyone around him, to a withdrawn, quiet little lad who only played with his toy vehicles or watched videos. His behaviour had grown more and more difficult with bouts of screaming becoming more and more frequent. He slept for an average of five hours each night. The following are indicative of effects experienced by the family:

- Jenny was particularly stressed and anxious about the changes in Thomas and the effects on his sisters. She was having difficulty sleeping and felt that routine household tasks were slipping. She felt she was no longer coping well.

- Richard would return from work to a disorganized house. He was concerned about Thomas's regression, but also anxious about the effects on Jenny and his two daughters.

- Thomas's siblings had become angry and resentful due to the impact of Thomas on their lives. They no longer invited friends to the house, nor played together in the same room as Thomas, nor wanted to participate in family outings.

- Jenny had seen the health visitor and the GP to discuss Thomas's difficulties but had been told not to worry as Thomas's behaviours were due to his coming out of the 'terrible twos'.

■ The family's social network had almost disappeared, apart from Jenny's parents who were a great source of support.

■ When Thomas was 3 years and 6 months, and soon due to begin primary school, it was agreed that a referral to a consultant paediatrician was needed for a detailed assessment. This was a great relief to Jenny, Richard and Jenny's parents.

■ Subsequently, Jenny and Richard became involved in a round of appointments, check-ups and tests for Thomas that took ten months overall and a considerable amount of organization. By this time the primary school had called Jenny and Richard into school on several occasions to discuss the difficulties they were experiencing with Thomas.

■ Eventually a diagnosis of 'autistic tendencies and behaviours' was given for Thomas and he was later transferred to a special school several miles away, to which he travelled in a taxi provided by the local authority.

The reality of illustrative example 8.1 should help practitioners to reflect on the issues arising for individual family members, and as each family member will have an impact on Thomas, then the need for considerations in this area should become clear. To provide effectively for Thomas, practitioners would need to consider and support the needs of the family members with advice, support, time, referrals to other agencies and access to information.

Chapter 3 explored issues of diagnosis and assessment and highlighted the difficulties of securing a thorough, multidisciplinary assessment of the child using their individual strengths and difficulties to inform that diagnosis. To tick items on a checklist will not provide an answer. Wing (1995) suggests:

> Diagnosis depends upon obtaining a detailed developmental history from the parents and a careful assessment of the child's skills and disabilities. Time taken to listen to the parents' story with attention and interest gives a real understanding of the child and helps to establish the foundation for a good relationship with the family. (p. 19)

The difficulties of discriminating between autistic spectrum disorders and allied conditions, some manifesting with similar characteristics, were also highlighted, concluding that there is a clear need for specialist expertise in autistic spectrum disorders on the part of the diagnosing professional. Research indicates that whilst there are many highly trained and skilled diagnosing professionals there are still others who lack the specific expertise needed to diagnose accurately. Clearly, this is a crucial issue for the future of the child and, therefore, the family.

The fact that differences occur across the country in the routes to diagnosis simply complicates the situation further for parents and professionals alike. The diagnosing professional may be a clinical psychologist, a consultant paediatrician or in some areas, a multidisciplinary team may be involved. Levels of expertise in autism may vary considerably as some professionals may focus their work purely on autistic spectrum disorders diagnoses, whilst others may have a more varied caseload covering many conditions.

Diagnostic instruments commonly used to support the diagnostic process were described, with the DSM-IV and the ICD-10 being most common. The CARS and the CHAT were also highlighted, with the latter, developed in the UK, being suitable for use with children aged between 18 and 42 months. The CHAT is a useful indicator of possible autism but it is not in itself a diagnostic instrument. A range of other diagnostic tools was identified with an overview of the key principles being offered to inform the reader.

Early years practitioners can best support the diagnostic process by submitting a range of their standard observations and assessments that are an essential part of the everyday working life of the setting. These can cover a range of situations and activities within the setting that can help complete the 'jigsaw picture' of the whole child. With the combination of these observations and assessments, the diagnostic assessment and detailed information gained from the parents, a more accurate diagnosis is likely.

Chapter 4 focused on practitioner understanding of the world of the child with autism. This knowledge is fundamental to effective provision as the characteristics and behaviours of young children with autism are very individual, but with some commonalities, and as such can be difficult to manage if practitioners are not fully aware of the implications. Awareness of issues surrounding the apparent unwillingness of young children with autism to participate in the range of activities that settings generally offer, will be crucial if adults are to respond appropriately.

Based on the triad of impairments, characteristics of an autistic spectrum disorder were explained in some detail with real examples used to illustrate and highlight specific points. This understanding should enable practitioners to relate the theoretical analyses to the practical realities of their working environment. My own experiences were offered to support the practitioner's perspective as it was considered that situations I had faced would be familiar to others working in early years settings. My own explanations and outcomes would hopefully inform the practice of others.

A particular focus was placed on understanding the sensory difficulties experienced by many young children with autism. Natural responses from any adults to young children in a range of situations may involve physical touch and contact, but for young children with autism experiencing sensory difficulties this might create physical pain and discomfort for the child, resulting in unexpected and unusual responses and behaviours. Again lack of understanding and awareness on the part of practitioners can thus compound the difficulties of the child, as opposed to the support that was intended. Sensory difficulties can also extend to hearing and sight, so typically noisy and visually stimulating early years settings can also create immediate difficulties for some children with autism, hence their covering of eyes and/or ears. As with many features and characteristics of any condition or disorder, once practitioners have the basic knowledge, then appropriate support can be devised which will be more likely to result in progress and positive achievements for the child.

This leads us back to the issues of training and funding which have emerged consistently throughout this book. Following on from this is the need for equity of access to training for all early years practitioners, not just those who are fortunate enough to be working in settings that are adequately funded and have the means to support the professional development of their staff. The preliminary findings of the small-scale research project offer more support as 51.55 per cent of all respondents indicated a desire to participate in autism training within the next academic year. To ensure that all early years practitioners have adequate levels of underpinning knowledge, this issue should be addressed as a matter of priority. Within the current inclusive climate we should not place expectations on staff that are unrealistic. Training must be made available to all, and preferably instigated at national level to ensure quality and consistency.

Chapter 5 examined a range of intervention programmes currently available to support young children with autism, but yet again we found that within any one local authority the range of specific approaches actually available to children will vary considerably, so the issue of equity arises again. The importance of early identification was highlighted which would hopefully lead to appropriate provision to support the child him/herself and the family members, but again we found that some parents had experienced considerable time lapses between diagnosis and access to provision. The issues of effective diagnoses and the subsequent availability of provision were highlighted as crucial success factors. Research evidence was offered to support the value and need for early identification, but within current legislation and guidance this view is already deemed essential (DfES, 2001b; DfES, 2001d; DfES, 2002; DfES/DoH, 2002; QCA, 2000). The need for effective and early identification is therefore now a requirement, yet as was highlighted previously, problems related to securing definitive diagnoses still exist and access to thorough and detailed diagnostic processes are not standard nationwide.

The most well-known specific approaches to autism, such as Lovaas, TEACCH and SPELL, were defined within Chapter 5 to extend practitioner knowledge and awareness, but were simply indicative of the wide range of approaches that currently exists and appears to expand with frequent regularity. Due to the comparative newness of some approaches there is little research evidence to indicate the success or otherwise of the approaches, but the more established approaches are generally well supported by research. The individual nature of each approach will, however, have a range of advocates and opponents, each with their own story to tell to support their claims. Parental decisions and choices will be crucial, but without adequate and accessible information they cannot necessarily make fully informed decisions. Having made their choice, parents may then discover that their preferred choice is unavailable within their own area and the local authority will not support the financing of access to the chosen setting. As long as the authority considers, and can justify, that the setting they do offer can provide effectively for the child, then parents may have great difficulty in securing an alternative.

It is not always appropriate or possible for an early years setting to support one specific approach, but it is more likely that settings will develop provision that incorporates aspects of several approaches, in an eclectic manner, which directly responds to the specific strengths and difficulties of the child. This was the case in my own working practice, as I used a basic TEACCH approach but supplemented the TEACCH strategies with elements from other approaches, including the sensory theory approach.

Chapter 6 continued to develop the theme of providing for young children with autism through exploring a range of strategies that would be likely to address the difficulties within the triad of impairments as opposed to adhering to one specific approach. This breakdown of strategies should offer practitioners clear and practical suggestions to develop within their own settings that will be based on their knowledge of the characteristics of autism, the implications for the setting and the planning of activities to promote and encourage success and progress for the individual child. Suggestions for appropriate planning and the use of IEPs, which inform planning and progress for the child and are reviewed regularly, were also examined. Without the underpinning knowledge offered in earlier chapters, future progress cannot be guaranteed. Issues of training, equity of access to training, funding and resources all resurface. However, even with the relevant knowledge, practitioners will need to be resourceful and flexible, which in my experience are characteristic of the majority of early years practitioners. The supporting strategies offered for each area of difficulty are not revolutionary in any respect, but reflect common strategies that will be familiar to most parents and practitioners. They were developed from knowledge of child development, experiences of providing for children with special needs and those with autism. The crucial factor regarding the selection and use of appropriate strategies is knowing the individual child and tailoring the strategies to meet that child's needs.

Chapter 7 began to explore the issue of inclusion and debated whether special or mainstream facilities could provide more appropriately for young children with autism. Historical developments in the field of inclusive provision were developed to place the discussions in context, which were followed by a consideration of the range of early years settings currently offering provision for children with autistic spectrum disorders. The research of Evans et al. (2001) evaluating current provision, was introduced to further develop discussions, and concluded that *placement* was less important than *expertise*. This supports the main premise of this book, which is that without knowledge and expertise in the field of autism, practitioners cannot, and should not be expected to, provide appropriately and effectively for young children with autism in mainstream settings. The research of Barnard, Prior and Potter (2000), which specifically focused on issues of inclusion and autism, further supports this premise when concluding that 'very few schools have staff who are adequately trained' (p. 7).

The speed of change within the fields of special needs provision and inclusion were also highlighted as fundamental issues for early years practitioners as a high percentage will be working on an hourly basis for near to the minimum wage. The expectation to read and interpret the considerable array of documentation that has been produced, particularly over the last five years, is considerable and, arguably, unacceptable for such practitioners. It could be suggested that to ensure the effectiveness of provision for young children with autism would require a nationwide training programme prior to the commencement of increased inclusion in mainstream settings. This would ensure that all early years practitioners would have the necessary underpinning knowledge with which to develop carefully planned, appropriate provision which could respond directly to the individual needs of the children and their families.

Throughout this book the key recurring issues have been:

■ training – appropriate and accessible to all practitioners;

■ funding – for training and resources;

■ resources – human and material;

■ equity of access to provision for children.

The recent Audit Commission report (2002a) adds further support to many of the emerging issues from this book. Whilst examining current SEN provision in the UK, the report focused on the four areas of identification, presence, participation and achievement. Key recommendations include the development of practitioner skills through an audit of training needs followed by a systematic programme of relevant training plus, 'the effective allocation and management of resources' (ibid., p. 56). The subsequent Audit Commission report (2002b) continued these themes by offering LEAs a handbook to support a self-evaluation of current SEN provision and to identify key issues within that authority that need addressing. Around the same time came the government's SEN Action Programme consultation document (Internet 11), suggesting ways forward within the field of SEN provision over the next ten years. The overall aim being that: 'all children with SEN and disabilities to realise their potential by improving access to education, raising standards of teaching and learning and strengthening partnerships with children, parents and carers' (Internet 11). The following areas were identified as key areas to be targeted, which again reflect some of the key themes within this book:

- early identification and early intervention;

- access to provision and inclusive practices;

- raising attainment levels and encouraging and supporting achievement;

- planning for stages of transition;

- multi-disciplinary working;

- monitoring and accountability.

Whilst there may appear to be some elements of negativity throughout the chapters of this book, it is related to a desire to ensure that young children with autism have access to high-quality early years settings that are staffed by skilled practitioners who are fully conversant with the issues surrounding the world of autism. Such staff would understand the characteristics of autism within the triad of impairments and be able to effectively observe and assess the young children they work with. This would in turn inform planning, leading to access to appropriate and stimulating activities that directly respond to the individual needs of the child, are likely to ensure success and build on previous achievements, and thus ensure continued progress. Each child will then be assured of working towards his/her full potential, at whatever level that might be. Issues of training, funding and resources combined with requirements on practitioners to assimilate information from regularly produced national documents are current obstacles to such an ideal. These issues are also linked to equity of access (to training and to provision), pay and equity within the early years field and lack of diagnostic coherence nationwide. Although there is evidence that provision for children with autism is certainly moving in the right direction we still have a way to go. Some young children with autistic spectrum disorders are attending settings that do not have the necessary expertise, knowledge and skills to provide appropriately for their individual needs and until such situations cease to exist then we still have work to do. At the end of the day young children with autism are simply young children, with rights, with needs, with desires and with concerns. They are entitled to equal opportunities and equal access to high-quality provision, so it is our responsibility to get it right.

Bibliography

Aarons, M. and Gittens, T. (1999) (2nd ed) *The Handbook of Autism: A Guide for Parents and Professionals*. 2nd edn. London: Routledge.

Adrien, J. L., Barthélémy, C., Perrot, A., Roux, S., Lenoir, P., Haumery, L. and Sauvage, D. (1992) 'Validity and reliability of the Infant Behavioural Summarized Evaluation (IBSE): a rating scale for the assessment of young children with autism and developmental disorders' *Journal of Autism and Developmental Disorders*, 22, pp. 375–94.

American Psychiatric Association (1994) *Diagnostic and Statistical Manual of Mental Disorders*, 4th edn. Washington, DC: American Psychological Association.

Attwood, T. (1998) *Asperger's Syndrome: A Guide for Parents and Professionals*. London: Jessica Kingsley.

Audit Commission (2002a) *SEN: A Mainstream Issue*. London: Audit Commission.

Audit Commission (2002b) *Managing Special Educational Needs: A Self-Review Handbook for Local Education Authorities*. London: Audit Commission.

Barnard, J., Prior, A. and Potter, D. (2000) *Inclusion and Autism: Is It Working?* London: NAS.

Barnes, P. (ed.) (1995) *Personal, Social and Emotional Development of Children*. Buckingham: Open University Press.

Baron-Cohen, S. and Bolton, P. (1993) *Autism: The Facts*. Oxford: Oxford University Press.

Baron-Cohen, S., Allen, J. and Gillberg, C. (1992) 'Can autism be detected at 18 months? The needle, the haystack and the CHAT', *British Journal of Psychiatry*, 161, pp. 839–43.

Barthélémy, C., Adrien, J. L., Roux, S., Garreau, B., Perrot, A. and LeLord, G. (1992) 'Sensitivity and specificity of the behavioural summarized evaluation for the assessment of autistic behaviours', *Journal of Autism and Developmental Disorders*, 22, pp. 23–31.

Beyer, B., and Gammeltoft, L. (2000) *Autism and Play*. London: Jessica Kingsley.

Bleuler, E. (1919) 'Das Autustisch – Undisziplinierte Denken in der Medizin und seine Ueberwindung'. Cited in L. Wing (ed.) (1976) *Early Childhood Autism*. 2nd edn. Oxford: Pergamon Press.

Carpenter, B. (1997) *Families in Context*. London: David Fulton.

Carpenter, B. (2000) 'Sustaining the family: meeting the needs of families of children with disabilities', *British Journal of Special Education*, 27(3), pp. 135–43.

Court, S.D.M. (1976) *Fit for the Future: The Report of the Committee on Child Health Services. Volume 1* (Court Report). London: HMSO.

Cumine, V., Leach, J. and Stephenson, G. (2000) *Autism in the Early Years: A Practical Guide*. London: David Fulton.

Dale, N. (1996) *Working with Families of Children with Special Needs*. London: Routledge.

Davies, J. (n.d.) *Children with Autism: A Booklet for Brothers and Sisters*. Nottingham: Child Development Research Unit, University of Nottingham.

Davis, B. (2001) *Breaking Autism's Barriers: A Father's Story*. London: Jessica Kingsley.

Department for Education and Employment (DfEE) (1993) *Education Act*. London: HMSO.

Department for Education and Employment (DfEE) (1994) *Code of Practice on the Identification and Assessment of Special Educational Needs*. London: HMSO.

Department for Education and Employment (DfEE) (1996) *Nursery Education and Grant Maintained Schools Act*. London: HMSO.

Department for Education and Skills (DfES) (2001a) *Special Educational Needs and Disability Discrimination Act 2001*. London: HMSO.

Department for Education and Skills (DfES) (2001b) *Special Educational Needs Code of Practice*. Nottingham: DfES.

Department for Education and Skills (DfES) (2001c) *Special Educational Needs Toolkit*. Nottingham: DfES.

Department for Education and Skills (DfES) (2001d) *Inclusive Schooling: Children with Special Educational Needs*. Nottingham: DfES.

Department for Education and Skills (DfES) (2001e) *Access to Education for Children and Young People with Medical Needs*. London: HMSO.

Department for Education and Skills (DfES) (2001f) *Access to Education for Children and Young People with Medical Needs*. Nottingham: DfES.

Department for Education and Skills (DfES) (2002) *Intervening Early*. Nottingham: DfES.

Department for Education and Skills/ Department of Health DfES/DoH. 2002. *Autistic Spectrum Disorders: Good Practice Guidance*. Nottingham: DfES.

Department of Education and Science (DES) (1970) *Education (Handicapped Children) Act*. London: HMSO.

Department of Education and Science (DES) (1978) *The Report of the Committee of Enquiry into the Education of Handicapped Children and Young People* (Warnock Report). London: HMSO.

Department of Education and Science (DES) (1981) *Education Act*. London: HMSO.

Department of Health (DoH) (1991) *The Children Act Guidance and Regulations. Volume 2: Family Support, Daycare and Educational Provision for Young Children*. London: HMSO.

DiLavore, P.C., Lord, C. and Rutter, M. (1995) 'The pre-linguistic autism diagnostic observation schedule', *Journal of Autism and Developmental Disorders*, 4, pp. 355–79.

Disability Rights Commission (DRC) (2001) *Draft Code of Practice (Schools)*. London: Disability Rights Commission.

Evans, J., Castle, F., Barraclough, S., and Jones, G. (2001) *Making a Difference: Early Interventions for Children with Autistic Spectrum Disorders*. Slough: NfER.

Freeman, B.J., Ritvo, E.R. and Schroth, P. (1984) 'Behaviour assessment of the syndrome of autism: behaviour observation system', *Journal of the American Academy of Child Psychiatry*, 23, pp. 588–94.

Freeman, B.J., Ritvo, E.R., Guthrie, D., Schroth, P. and Ball, J. (1978) 'The behaviour observation scale for autism: initial methodology, data analysis and preliminary findings on 89 children', *Journal of the American Academy of Child Psychiatry*, 17, pp. 576–88.

Gillingham, G. (1995) *Autism. Handle with Care!* Texas: Future Horizons.

Gorrod, L. (1997) *My Brother Is Different*. London: NAS.

Harris, S. (1994) *Siblings of Children with Autism*. Bethesda: Woodbine.

Herbert, E. and Carpenter, B. (1994) 'Fathers – the secondary partners: professional perceptions and a father's reflections', *Children and Society*, 8(1), 31–41.

Howlin, P. (1998) *Children with Autism and Asperger Syndrome: A Guide for Practitioners and Carers*. Chichester: Wiley.

Howlin, P. and Moore, A. (1997) 'Diagnosis in autism: a survey of over 1200 patients', *Autism: The International Journal of Research and Practice*. 1, 135–62.

Jones, G. (2002) *Educational Provision for Children with Autism and Asperger Syndrome. Meeting their Needs*. London: David Fulton.

Jordan, R. and Libby, S. (1997) 'Developing and using play in the curriculum', in S. Powell and R. Jordan (eds), *Austism and Learning: A Guide to Good Practice*. London: David Fulton.

Jordan, R., Jones, G. and Murray, D. (1998) *Educational Interventions for Children with Autism: A Literature Review of Recent and Current Research*. Sudbury: DfEE.

Kanner, L. (1943) 'Autistic disturbances of affective contact'. *Nervous Child*, 2, pp. 217–50.

Krug, D. A., Arick, J. and Almond, P. (1980) 'Behaviour checklist for identifying severely handicapped individuals with high levels of autistic behaviour', *Journal of Autism and Developmental Disorders*. 18, pp. 647–56.

Le Couter, A., Rutter, N., Lord, C., Rios, P., Robertson, S., Holdgrafter, M. and McLennen, J.D. (1989) 'Autism Diagnostic Interview: a standardized, investigator-based instrument', *Journal of Autism and Developmental Disorders*, 19, pp. 363–87.

Leicestershire County Council and Fosse Health Trust (1998) *Autism – How to Help your Young Child*. London: National Autistic Society.

Lotter, V. (1967) *The Prevalence of the Autistic Syndrome in Children*. London: University of London Press.

Lord, C., Rutter, M. Goode, S., Heemsberger, J., Jordan, M. Mawhood, L. and Schopler, E. (1989) 'Autism diagnostic observations schedule: a standardized observation of communicative and social behaviour', *Journal of Autism and Development Disorders*, 19, pp. 185–212.

Ministry of Education (1944) *Education Act*. London: HMSO.

Murray, D. (1997) 'Autism and information technology: therapy with computers', in S. Powell and R. Jordan (eds), *Autism and Learning. A guide to good practice*. London: David Fulton.

National Autistic Society (NAS) (1999a) *Diagnosis – Reactions in Families*. London: National Autistic Society.

National Autistic Society (NAS) (1999b). *Opening the Door: A Report on Diagnosis and Assessment of Autism and Asperger Syndrome Based on Personal Experiences*. London: National Autistic Society.

National Austistic Society (NAS) (2000) *Experience of the whole family*. London: NAS.

National Autistic Society (2001) *Approaches to Autism*. London: National Autistic Society.

National Foundation for Educational Research (2001) *Making a Difference: Early Interventions for Children with Austistic Spectrum Disorders*. Slough: NfER.

Peeters, T. (1997) *Autism: From Theoretical Understanding to Educational Intervention*. London: Whurr Publishers.

Powell, S. and Jordan, R. (eds) (1997) *Autism and Learning: A Guide to Good Practice*. London: David Fulton.

Pugh, G. (ed.) (2001) *Contemporary Issues in the Early Years*, 3rd edn. London: Paul Chapman Publishing.

Qualifications and Curriculum Authority (QCA) (1999) *Early Learning Goals*. London: QCA.

Qualifications and Curriculum Authority (QCA) (2000) *Curriculum Guidance for the Foundation Stage*. London: QCA.

Reichler, R.J. and Schopler, E. (1971) 'Observations on the nature of human relatedness', *Journal of Autism and Childhood Schizophrenia*. 1, pp. 283–96.

Rimland, B. (1971) 'The differentiation of childhood psychoses: an analysis of checklists for 2, 218 psychotic children', *Journal of Autism and Childhood Schizophrenia*, 1, 161–74.

Rutter, M. and Schopler, E. (eds) (1978) *Autism*. New York: Plenum Press.

Rutter, M., LeCouter, A., Lord, C., MacDonald, H., Rios, P. and Folstein, S. (1988) 'Diagnosis and subclassification of autism: Concepts and instrument development', in E. Schopler, E. and G. Mesibov (eds), *Diagnosis and Assessment in Autism*. New York: Plenum Press.

Schopler, E., Reichler, R.J., and Renner, B.R. (1986) *The Childhood Autism Rating Scale (CARS)*. Los Angeles: Western Psychological Services.

Schopler, E., Reichler, R.J., DeVellis, R.F. and Daly, K. (1980) 'Toward objective classification of childhood autism: Childhood Autism Rating Scale (CARS)', *Journal of Autism and Developmental Disorders*, 10, 91–103.

Seach, D. (1998) *Autistic Spectrum Disorders: Positive approaches for teaching children with ASD*. London: NASEN.

Siegel, B. (1996) *The World of the Autistic Child: Understanding and Treating Autistic Spectrum Disorders*. Oxford: Oxford University Press.

Shields, J. (2000) 'The NAS Early Bird Programme: autism-specific early intervention for parents', *Professional Care of Mother and Child*, 10, (2), pp. 53–4.

Trevarthen, C., Aitken, K., Papoudi, D., and Robarts, J. (1998) *Children with Autism: Diagnosis and Interventions to Meet their Needs*. London: Jessica Kingsley.

Wall, K. (2003a) *Special Needs and Early Years: A Practitioner's Guide*. London: Sage.

Wall, K. (2003b) 'The golden rule is that the family must come first', *Early Years Educator*, 5(6), 62–4.

Wing, L. (ed.) (1976) *Early Childhood Autism*. 2nd edn. Oxford: Pergamon Press.

Wing, L. (1995) *Autistic Spectrum Disorders: An Aid to Diagnosis*. London: National Autistic Society.

Wing, L. and Gould, J. (1978) 'Systematic recording of behaviours and skills of retarded and psychotic children', *Journal of Autism and Childhood Schizophrenia*, 8, pp. 79–97.

World Health Organization (WHO) (1993) *International Classification of Diseases, Tenth Revision*. Geneva: WHO.

Internet sites

Internet 1:   www.dfes.gov.uk (accessed 18.10.2002).

Internet 2:   www.teacch.com/20ques (accessed: 03.02.2002).

Internet 3:   www.bobjanet.demon.co.uk/lks (accessed: 18.06.2003).

Internet 4:   wwww.williams-syndrome.org/forparents/whatiswilliams (accessed: 18.04.2003).

Internet 5:   www.pwsausa.org/syndrome/index (accessed: 10.06.2003).

Internet 6:   www.fragilex.org/what (accessed 18.06.2003).

Internet 7:   www.nas.org.uk (accessed 06.03.2000).

Internet 8:   www.autism.org/temple/inside (accessed 09.05.2001).

Internet 9:   www.mrc.ac.uk (accessed 12.08.2003).

Internet 10:   www.nas.org.uk/ (accessed 11.08.2003).

Internet 11:   www.dfes.gov.uk/sen/documents (accessed 09.09.2003).

Index

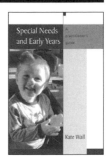